10. Coconut Oil: Why

    http://www.coconut

11. Chlorella benefits and information:

    http://www.herbwisdom.com/herb-chlorella.html

12. Heinerman, John. *Encyclopedia of Healing Juices*. West

    Nyack, NY. Parker Publishing Co., 1994.

    (www.betterway2health.com)

Recipe Resources:

http://www.glutenfreeda.com

http://www.cooks.com/

http://allrecipes.com/

http://www.internationalrecipesonline.com

http://www.recipe-source.com/

http://www.stgabriel.net/stgabriel_new/school/international_reci

pes.htm

Kolkata, India; Central Institute for Research (Ayurveda), Kolkata, India. <u>The Role of Iron Chelation Activity of Wheat Grass Juice in Patients with Myelo-dysplastic Syndrome</u>. *Journal of Clinical Oncology* 27:15s, 2009 (suppl; abstr 7012) 2009 ASCO Annual Meeting. Presenter:Soma Mukhopadhyay, PhD.

4. <u>Fatal Diseases Related to Inflammation</u>: www.leveldiet.com © 2010 Level1Diet.com

5. <u>Grain Information</u>: www. Aaoobfoods.com. Copyright © 2000 AAOOB Products (Revised July 2009)

6. The Glycemic Index. www.high-fiber-health.com. Copyright 2004-2008 High-Fiber-Health.com

7. <u>The Acid-Alkaline Diet</u>. http://acidalkalinediet.com/Alkaline-Foods-Chart.htm

8. <u>Anti-inflammatory Food</u>. http://www.metabolismadvice.com/anti_inflammatory_food/

9. <u>The Benefits of Coconut Oil</u> http://www.organicfacts.net/organic-oils/organic-coconut-oil/health-benefits-of-coconut-oil.htm

Eat Your Disease Away

Maiysha T Clairborne MD

Atlanta, GA USA

ISBN 1453615067

Printed in the United States of America.

Preface

This book is a guide to fighting inflammatory diseases, fibromyalgia, chronic fatigue syndrome, polymyalgia, lupus and other autoimmune based disorders. In this book we will be exploring what foods cause inflammation, why preparation method is so important, and how to use the anti-inflammatory diet to change the course of any inflammatory disease. We will also explore healthy detoxification and supplements that I consider essential to cleansing and to every day health and well-being. Next, we will take the journey through the processes of healthy shopping, meal planning, healthy cooking basics, and quick preparation for the busy person. Finally you will learn simple, fun, and practical tips that you can incorporate into an efficient daily practice through meal planning. By the end of this book you will understand the body's inflammatory process, know how to use food to reverse this, and realize that it doesn't have to be overwhelming, stressful, or expensive, and that it can in fact be quite simple, tasty, cost effective and even fun.

EAT YOUR DISEASE AWAY

Table of Contents

1

Introduction: The Body and Inflammation

Inflammation is the constant irritation of the body's cells. Imagine constantly being emotionally irritated all the time. Imagine someone poking you for 24 hours a day, seven days a week. That's irritating. Now, imagine what effect that would have on your mental state. The same effect applies to the body. Imagine every cell in your body constantly irritated, 24-7. This is the effect that inflammation has on the body. This kind of injury leads to chemical cascade, which can lead to formation of all types of diseases, including

Fibromyalgia

Lupus

Chronic fatigue

Thyroid diseases such as Graves and Hashimotos

Candida or yeast overgrowth

1

Inflammation can also cause high blood sugars high blood pressure, and elevated cholesterol, which lead to other complications such as heart attack, stroke, and many other problems. The bottom line is that poor dietary and lifestyle choices lead to this inflammation, thereby causing the injury and disease to occur, and that through shifting to a more alkaline and less inflammatory diet, we can halt and even reverse the causes of these diseases.

Let's talk about acid versus alkaline. The optimal Ph of the body in a healthy state is between 8 and 9. This is when the body functions most efficiently. But when the body becomes more acid in nature, the cells become inflamed and the doors are open for abnormal cell function that lead to disease. So what are some of the inflammatory and non-inflammatory foods? I have compiled a list of both Non-Inflammatory, Neutral and Inflammatory foods by food type in the charts below. Which foods do you find more in your pantry or refrigerator?

Chart 1: Anti-Inflammatory Foods Chart

Vegetables	Fruits
Garlic	Apples
Asparagus	Apricot
Beets	Avocado (yes, avocado is a
Broccoli	fruit)
Cabbage	Bananas
Carrot	Cherries
Cauliflower	Grapefruit (which may be
Celery	acidic in nature but is alkalizing
Collard greens	to the body)
Cucumber	Lime
Eggplant	Oranges
Kale	Lemons
Lettuce	Peaches
Mushrooms	Pears
Mustard greens	Pineapples
Peas	All berries
Peppers	Tomatoes
Onions	Watermelon (which is also
Rutabagas	very cleansing in nature)
Pumpkins	
Peppers	
Alfalfa grass	

Wheat and barley grass Wild greens	
Oriental Vegetables	**Grains**
Maitaki mushrooms	Amaranth
Shitake mushrooms	Barley
Reishi mushrooms	Buckwheat
Wakami	Oats
Sea vegetables	Quinoa
Dandelion root	Rye
Daikon	Spelt
	Camlet
	Hemp seed flours
Seasonings include:	**Other Foods/Seasonings Etc**
Cinnamon	Probiotic cultures
Curries	Vegetable juices
Ginger	Mineral water
Mustard	Green tea and other herbal teas
Chili peppers	Ginseng tea
Sea salt	Campeche tea
Miso	
All herbs	
Tamari	
Stevia sweetener	

Chart 2: Neutral Foods (In Moderation)

Legumes	Grains
Black beans	Oats
Chickpeas,	All rices
Green peas,	Rye
Kidney beans,	Spelt
Lentils,	Camlet
Pinto beans,	Wheat
Red beans,	
Soy beans,	
Soy milk,	
White beans,	
Almond milk	
Proteins	**Other Foods/Seasonings Etc**
Whey protein powder	Apple cider vinegar
Some cottage cheeses	Avocado oil
Eggs	Hemp seed
Almonds	Flax oil
Some tofu that's fermented	Ghee
Pumpkin seeds	Olive oil
Tempe (which is a fer-	Sucranat / Cane Sugar

mented type of soy product that's often used in place of meant) Other nuts and sprouted seed	Maple Syrup (Grade A or B) Agave Nectar

Chart 3: Inflammatory Foods

Meats/Protein	Fats & Oils
Beef Clams Fish Lamb Lobster Mussels Oyster Pork Rabbit Salmon Shrimp Scallops Tuna Turkey Venison	Canola oil Canola Corn Lard Sesame Safflower oil

Dairy	Other foods/spices/etc
Milk	White Sugar
Cheese	Brown Sugar
Butter	Corn Syrup
Ice Cream	Chemicals
Heavy Cream	Medicinal
Eggs	Pesticides
Organic, unpasteurized milk	Herbicides
	Alcohol (all alcohol)

When we talk about the acid versus the alkaline diet, most people should have a 60-40 split. That's 60% alkaline and 40% acidic. Now, if you're doing a hardcore cleanse then you might want to go more 80-20, and if you have one of the diseases like fibromyalgia or lupus or any autoimmune, again, you want to think about going 80% alkaline and 20% acidic.

Now let's talk a little bit about food combining. When you talk about food combining, the importance of this is so that the food that you eat is properly digested and absorbed into the body. So let's start with your fruits. Acid fruits, such as grape-fruits, lemons, limes, oranges, pineapples, pomegranates, strawberries, tangerines and tomatoes are best combined with your sub-acid fruits. Those are apples, apricots, berries, cherries, grapes, fresh figs, kiwi, mango, nectarine, papaya, pears, and plums. And your sub-acid fruits, in addition to being combined with acid fruits, can also be combined with your sweet fruits. Those are your bananas, coconuts, dates, figs, persimmons, raisins, and dry fruits. Your sweet fruits should not be combined with your acid fruits. And melons, like your cantaloupes, honeydews, watermelon, they should be eaten alone and not combined with any other fruit.

Now let's go on to vegetables, proteins and starches. Generally, proteins can be combined with low- and non-starchy vegetables, so for example, your dry beans or tofu or peanuts may be combined with a non- or low-starchy vegetable such as asparagus, beets, broccoli, carrots, peppers, scallions, spinach, or any leafy green, and your low-and non-starchy vegetables can be combined with your carbohydrate starches, such as bread, other dry beans, pastas, potatoes, and yams.

Generally, protein and starchy carbohydrates are not good combinations. Neither are proteins or starchy carbohydrates with fats such as avocado oils, corn oil, olive oil, Safire oil, or even olives, coconuts, and avocados. Your low- and non-starchy vegetables can be combined with fats, such as your avocados, coconut, or olives, so you might make a salad, a spinach salad, with broccoli and radish, scallions, peppers, and a leafy green and combine it with avocado and maybe a vinegar and oil dressing. I've included a chart so that you can see all of this at a glance. (See chart 3)

Chart3: Food Combining

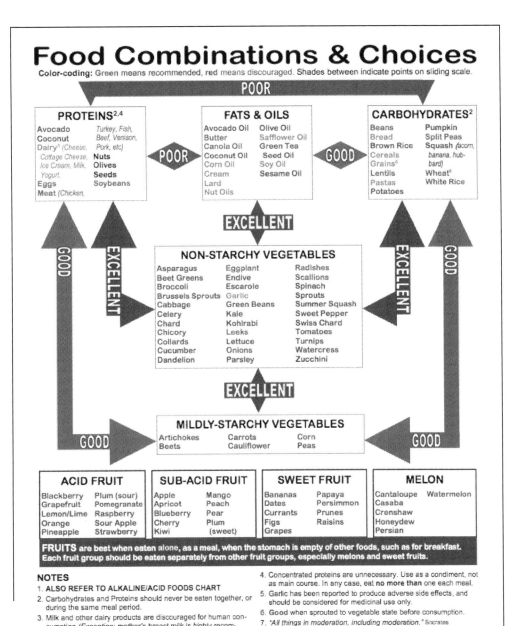

Food Combinations & Choices

Color-coding: Green means recommended, red means discouraged. Shades between indicate points on sliding scale.

POOR

PROTEINS[2,4]

Avocado	Turkey, Fish,
Coconut	Beef, Venison,
Dairy³ (Cheese,	Pork, etc)
Cottage Cheese,	**Nuts**
Ice Cream, Milk,	**Olives**
Yogurt,	**Seeds**
Eggs	**Soybeans**
Meat (Chicken,	

POOR

FATS & OILS

Avocado Oil	Olive Oil
Butter	Safflower Oil
Canola Oil	Green Tea
Coconut Oil	Seed Oil
Corn Oil	Soy Oil
Cream	Sesame Oil
Lard	
Nut Oils	

GOOD

CARBOHYDRATES[2]

Beans	Pumpkin
Bread	Split Peas
Brown Rice	Squash (acorn,
Cereals	banana, hub-
Grains⁶	bard)
Lentils	Wheat⁶
Pastas	White Rice
Potatoes	

EXCELLENT

NON-STARCHY VEGETABLES

Asparagus	Eggplant	Radishes
Beet Greens	Endive	Scallions
Broccoli	Escarole	Spinach
Brussels Sprouts	Garlic	Sprouts
Cabbage	Green Beans	Summer Squash
Celery	Kale	Sweet Pepper
Chard	Kohlrabi	Swiss Chard
Chicory	Leeks	Tomatoes
Collards	Lettuce	Turnips
Cucumber	Onions	Watercress
Dandelion	Parsley	Zucchini

GOOD · EXCELLENT · EXCELLENT · GOOD

EXCELLENT

MILDLY-STARCHY VEGETABLES

Artichokes	Carrots	Corn
Beets	Cauliflower	Peas

GOOD · GOOD

ACID FRUIT

Blackberry	Plum (sour)
Grapefruit	Pomegranate
Lemon/Lime	Raspberry
Orange	Sour Apple
Pineapple	Strawberry

SUB-ACID FRUIT

Apple	Mango
Apricot	Peach
Blueberry	Pear
Cherry	Plum
Kiwi	(sweet)

SWEET FRUIT

Bananas	Papaya
Dates	Persimmon
Currants	Prunes
Figs	Raisins
Grapes	

MELON

Cantaloupe	Watermelon
Casaba	
Crenshaw	
Honeydew	
Persian	

FRUITS are best when eaten alone, as a meal, when the stomach is empty of other foods, such as for breakfast. Each fruit group should be eaten separately from other fruit groups, especially melons and sweet fruits.

NOTES

1. ALSO REFER TO ALKALINE/ACID FOODS CHART
2. Carbohydrates and Proteins should never be eaten together, or during the same meal period.
3. Milk and other dairy products are discouraged for human consumption (Exception: mother's breast milk is highly recommended for babies of the same species!)
4. Concentrated proteins are unnecessary. Use as a condiment, not as main course. In any case, eat no more than one each meal.
5. Garlic has been reported to produce adverse side effects, and should be considered for medicinal use only.
6. Good when sprouted to vegetable state before consumption.
7. "All things in moderation, including moderation." Socrates
8. This information may be copied and distributed freely.

Now that we've talked a little bit about food combining, let's just go over the basics of healthy eating. One of the main important things about healthy eating is how much to eat and how often to eat. Let's talk about portions first. This is kind of the easy part. In the US our portions are way too big. If you go to a restaurant they give you these huge portions. Later on in this series we'll talk about a couple of tips to minimize or to get the most out of restaurant eating. However, let's get back to portions. Generally, if you take a regular sized dinner plate and divide it into four, one-quarter of that should be for starch, one-quarter for meat and one-half for vegetables. Keep in mind that there is no need to go for seconds.

Now let's talk about how often. Generally we eat two or three meals a day as Americans. We've gotten to this bad habit that less is more, but then when we do eat we're so hungry because we haven't eaten all day that we engorge ourselves. Here's what should happen: three major meals and two small snacks. So that's actually five small meals a day. The reason that eating five small meals a day is healthier is for several reasons. First, our body is made to graze and when we're constantly eating we're actually constantly burning energy. It does take calories to digest food, so it's important in maintaining weight. It's also important in maintaining metabolism. If you eat rarely then, when you do eat, your body tends to hold on to every little calorie – even the unhealthy ones. So that's another reason why five small meals are better than two huge, humungous meals. The third reason is that when you're eating small and more frequent meals, it's helping to normalize or keep your body from having these up-and-down insulin bursts. In essence, it helps to maintain your blood sugar. So just those three reasons alone should be enough to convince you that eating five small meals is better than just eating one or two large meals a day.

Some may ask, "How am I supposed to be get in five small meals a day?" That's three major meals and two snacks and it's absolutely do-able. We'll talk about this more, later.

What are the servings should you be getting? The answer is four to six servings of vegetables, three to four servings of fruit, 25 – 30 grams of protein, and 25 grams of fiber. What does that translate to? It translates to 2-3 vegetables, per meal, per day – including breakfast, two fruits at breakfast and maybe one for a snack, a fiber source and a protein source at each meal. Later we'll talk about how to get all of these servings of fruit, vegetable, protein and fibre into every meal. This will come in the Healthy Cooking section as well as the Six Small Meals section.

2

Detoxification & Cleansing

We've broken down a little bit about the body and inflammation and the basics of nutrition. Let's talk a little bit about detoxification and cleansing. There are so many products out there these days for detox and cleansing and even the word "detoxification' has become a buzzword in our society. But what really is detoxification and cleansing? Well, many of the things that we eat, even the air that we breathe, contain different toxins in them – such as pesticides, or we have pollutant in the air. These things, when we breathe them in or when we ingest them, they actually become absorbed into the body's system. Due to our standard American diet, a lot of times our body gets clogged up and is not able to properly eliminate the toxins that we take in on a daily basis. Occasionally, it's necessary to do a good, cleansing diet along with herbs that support the body's organ systems to mobilize and then to eliminate the toxins that we take in on a daily basis.

So, what are the systems that we're actually cleaning out when we do a full detox? Well, of course, it is important to keep our colon cleansed. We ingest things through our mouth, it goes through our intestinal system and is ingested – and the junk that's leftover is eliminated through our colon. So it's important to keep the large intestine functional so that we can eliminate on a daily basis the toxins that we're coming across as we eat these different foods. Another system that needs to be detoxified is the liver, as well as the kidneys. The liver is an organ that, when we digest and absorb certain nutrients and toxins into the body, the liver is one of the first lines of detoxifying organs. The liver neutralizes and helps to eliminate many of the toxins that we take in from medications and from certain foods. The kidneys are another important elimination system. Once some of the toxins have been neutralize din other organ systems, we elimi- nate a lot of unnecessary metabolites through the urine of the kidneys. As you can see, the two elimination systems that are most important are our colon and our kidney. Of course, we can't forget about the skin as a detoxifying organ.

Sweat is another way that we actually get rid of toxins out of the body. So with that said, there are several different ways to cleanse. When we talk about cleansing from the inside out, there are specific things that you can do in order to assist the body in its detoxifying and elimination process. One of those is the diet, and by conforming to either a raw food or an anti-inflammatory diet, which we just talked about, this helps the body to properly digest and eliminate food in the way that it is supposed to, at the same time building the body with the proper nutrients needed for the body to be able to heal itself. In terms of colon cleansing, there are several different methods to utilize. One is colon hydro cleansing also known as colonics. This is when water is inserted into the colon and the colon is literally washed out. It's a minimally invasive procedure that's done by trained professionals and can often increase energy and yield great results. It can help with constipation and it can also help with some malabsorption because a lot of times, if your colon system is clogged with junk that's been on the lining of the colon for many years, once you eliminate that, your body is better able to function, moving the excrement out of the system like it's intended to do.

The other organs that need to properly be detoxified are the lymph system and the blood, as well as the lungs. A great way to go about detoxifying the respiratory system is through deep breathing exercises. In another book of mine, Life On Your Terms, mindfulness is step two in coming to be more empowered and living a more healthy life. In these we talk about deep breathing exercises as not only a source of relaxation but as a source of delivering oxygen properly to the organs and eliminating respiratory toxins.

Detoxifying the blood and lymph system can be done through diet alone, but also there are many herbal products out there that can help to support the lymphatic and the blood system, mobilizing the toxins from each of these systems and dumping it into the renal system so that it can be eliminated through the urine.

When you're looking at herbal products for detoxification, you want to look at the company's reputation for creating quality herbal products that have been standardized. One great brand is RenewLife, also called Advance Naturals. This usually can be bought at your local Whole Foods. This is an herbal product that contains the herbs to support all of the organ systems including the liver, the kidney, the blood, the lymph, and the respiratory system. You take this for a period of either two weeks or four weeks and you along with a detoxifying diet and juicing, can get a very good cleanse in.

It's also important to know that cleansing, if overdone, can be dangerous. Detox and cleansing for long periods of time can break down the body more than it's supposed to be broken down. There are two components when you're detoxifying and cleansing the body. One is the actual breakdown of the toxins in elimination process, and the other is the building back up, so the body can heal and be healthy. If you're always detoxifying the colon or taking an herbal cleanse, you're only breaking down and mobilizing toxins and you're not building. If you detox with herbs alone, without the diet, all you're doing is wasting your money, because if you're still eating crap but then you're trying to detox, you're cancelling the whole process out. This is why it's important when you want to cleanse or detox, to do this under the supervision of a trained professional because then you can get the proper instruction on detox diet and you can get the most reliable products that will help your system to mobilize all of the toxins necessary in a safe manner.

How often should you detox? I've heard of people who have detoxed continuously throughout the year but again, that can be unsafe. It's overdoing it. Generally, a good long detox (meaning a four-week detox) should be done no more than twice a year. Once a year can even be sufficient if you normally have a pretty healthy living existence. But you can also do many cleanses throughout the year. No more than quarterly is necessary. So if you want to do a cleanse during the spring equinox, the summer solstice, the fall equinox and the winter solstice, those are great times, transitional times even, to do a detox for the body. And in terms of a long detox, once a year is sufficient.

Now that we've covered the basics of detox and cleansing, know that the diet that goes with detox and cleansing has been discussed in the anti-inflammatory section of this book, and the specifics of shopping and cooking for detox will be covered in the future chapters.

The Skinny on the Different Types of Cleanses
Today detox and cleansing has become a buzz word, a fad, and as such there are dozens of different so called "cleanses" out there. The purpose of a cleanse is to rid the body of toxins that have built up from years of improper dietary habits. In addition, a cleanse should be jump start to a lifestyle change (or back into your healthy lifestyle if you've fallen away from your normal healthy regimen). Today, many weight obsessed people use cleansing as a "quick fix" to lose weight. While weight loss can be a side effect of cleansing, it is not it's main purpose. Below, I will go over a few of them, their benefits and risks. Then I will tell you what a proper cleanse should look like and how often a person needs to cleanse. Finally, I will give you a couple of supplements that will augment your detox. First, let's start with a few cleanses that are out there:

1. Master Cleanser – This cleanse has been around for decades and has been modified and commercialized to some extent. Some call it the "lemonade diet". This cleanse consists of fasting for up to 10 days (for some up to 2-3 weeks), only taking in a juice comprised of lemon juice, cayenne pepper, grade A Maple syrup, and water. It is

said that the lemon juice and cayenne pepper is detoxifying, and the Maple syrup provides the nutrients. Typically, this cleanse is started by drinking 8 ounces of raw sea salt water to cleanse the colon. For a short term cleanse (2-3 days), this is not a bad endeavor, but fasting for long periods of time can slow the metabolism, lead to muscle wasting and nutrient deficiency, and for some can be dangerous for the health. People with diabetes or low blood sugar are not suited for this type of cleanse, and those with high blood pressure should be cautious, as while most of the salt is not absorbed, drinking sea salt water can drive the blood pressure up (some times to dangerous levels). Other so called "detoxes" similar to this are the "watermelon fast", "grapefruit diet", and juice fasting which will be discussed later on. While watermelon and grapefruit are great cleansing fruits, utilizing them alone as a cleanse does not constitute a thorough detox. At best you are simply diuresing (getting rid of excess water) and illuding yourself into think this is real weight loss.

2. Raw Food Cleanse: This cleanse is exactly what it sounds like. For 21-28 days, you eat only raw foods (fruits, vegetables, nuts, soaked and/or sprouted grains

prepared or unprepared). For many this cleanse can be extraordinary since most Americans partake of such poor diets. Just transitioning to a diet rich in fruits and vegetables while devoid of refined and overly processed foods, sugars, fats, and meats makes a significant difference in the physical well being of any person. There are many diseases that can be improved or healed by partaking this type of diet. However, long term this cleanse can actually put a strain on the digestive system, as raw foods are more difficult to digest. While I am not suggesting that overcooked foods are better, I am simply saying the finding a medium between raw and high heat cooked foods is probably best for long term health of the digestive system. More on that in the Healthy Cooking chapter.

3. Juice Fasting: Juice fasting is similar to the Master Cleanse in that it is an all liquid diet, but in reality, juice fasting (if done correctly) an be maintained slightly longer than the "Lemonade diet". This is vegetable juice is more dense and has more caloric value than the "juice" of the Master Cleanse. Take for instance a juice of combined spinach, carrot, apple, and celery; In this juice you will get several vitamins including Vitamins A, B, C,

Beta Carotene, and minerals such as calcium, magnesium, and zinc. The density of vegetable juice also has more sustenance than that of the Lemon concoction of the Master Cleanse. So, theoretically, one could juice fast for weeks and maintain their nutritional status. Obviously, however, it is unrealistic that most Americans will maintain this type of eating regimen for long term, and thus should be considered a short term cleanse solution. Perhaps a cleanse such as this is suited for quarterly use and for no longer than 1 week.

4. Colon cleansing: While the most important part of a cleanse is the cleansing of the digestive tract, it is not the only aspect of the cleanse. These days the world is focused on colon cleansing, and so much so that there are several different products masking as colon cleansers when they really are herbal laxatives. The problem with over-doing colon cleanses is two things: 1. People are so obsessed with using colon cleansing as a way to lose weight, that these "colon cleansing" products have a hight abuse rate and often can lead to purging (which by the way is a symptom of bulimia). 2. If overused, the herbal laxatives (like regular laxatives) can handicap the bowel such that when taken off of these products, the

.

bowel will not empty properly leading to functional constipation (due to low motility). There are several ways to colon cleanse ranging from colonics to herbs and powders. The most appropriate way to utilize the colon cleanse is in conjunction with a full organ detox. My personal recommendation is to start your cleanse out with colon hydrotherapy and continue on with a 14-21 day organ detox utilizing the eliminative diet that I will describe next.

The proper way to detox

As I previously alluded to, there are safe ways to detox. I use the word "safe" in plural, because there is more than one safe way to cleanse. It's not always which cleanse you choose, it's the understanding of how to utilize cleansing to better your health and well-being.   As important is the motivation for doing a detox program, how long and how often the cleansing program occurs.

There are two components or phases to a cleanse. The first is to break down, mobilize, and eliminate toxins from the body. The second is to build the body back up after the breakdown that the toxins has caused. This includes building the immune system and replenishing of nutrients that may have been deficient before the cleanse or even lost during the first phase of the cleanse.   It is important to include both of these components in a detox program otherwise you defeat the purpose of doing a "detox" in the first place. If there is detoxification without building, there is cell damage from toxins and free radicals caused by the toxins. This can lead to further illness and even cell mutation in the long run. Prolonged fasting has the same effect. This is the reason cleanses like the Master Cleanse or certain juice fasting should not be done for periods of time longer than one week. It's also the reason that long detox programs (21-28 days) should not be done more than twice a year. As a matter of fact, if the cleansing process is done properly, and the eating habits are maintained in a healthy way, there is no need to detox more than once a year. Of course, short cleanses (2-3 days) may be done quarterly if desired as a way to transition into each season, but this has more of a spiritual significance than a physical one.

Eating During the Detox

Probably the easiest and most sustainable type of diet to eat while on a detox is an eliminative diet. An eliminative diet simply means eliminating all of the things that cause inflammation are and build toxins. Now, this may sound simple (and it is), but for some it can be very challenging if you are used to eating fast foods, refined bleached products, fried foods, and junk snacks. When cleansing it is important to eliminate all of those things

23

mentioned in chapter one as inflammatory including sugar, meat, alcohol, refined grains and pasta, fried foods, and dairy to name a few. The key in this type of detox is to replace the things that you eliminate with a nutrional source that is anti-inflammatory and comparable. For example, if you are eliminating milk, you may consider replacing it with Almond Milk, Coconut Milk or Hemp Milk. Similarly, if you are eliminating white pasta and rice, you may substitute grains such as quinoa, amaranth, brown or wild rice. If you are giving up coffee for the cleanse, you might replace that with an herbal tea such as Chinese green, white, or Oolong tea. In eliminating meat, you will want to re-place your protein source using things like Seitan (unless you are gluten allergic), Tempeh, beans, lentils, chickpeas, or even nuts such as almonds or brazil nuts. You may used prepared deriva-tives such a hummus. The idea is that though you are eliminating several unhealthy foods from you diet, you will not go hungry because you will be replacing them with some healthy and rather tasty substitutes. How to prepare some of these new healthy foods will be covered in the Healthy Cooking chapter. The important thing to remember is that a cleanse should not leave you weak and listless. You may feel a bit tired the first week as your body mobilizes the toxins from the tissues and be-gins to eliminate them, but if you are feeling starved throughout the cleanse, you arenot eating enough. In addition, great caution should be taken for people with co-existing conditions such as diabetes, heart disease, low blood sugar, cancer, sickle cell, lupus, and other major health problems. If enough nutrients, water, or oxygen does not get to the system due to too low intake, it could cause crisis of the disease itself.

The final important thing to remember about detox eating is to hydrate appropriately. As stated earlier the colon, and kidneys are the main organs that rid the body of toxins. If you are taking supplements to mobilize the toxins but are not drinking enough water so that the kidneys and colon can properly eliminate them, you put yourself at risk for what's called a healing crisis. This is a result of the toxins floating around in the bloodstream. In a relatively healthy person the symptoms may be limited to headache, nausea, weakness, and fatigue. However, in those with co-morbid conditions the symptoms and consequences can be much more severe. When doing a detox program at least 2 liters of water should be taken daily unless you contain a condition that requires water restriction such as congestive heart failure or end stage kidney disease. In all cases, you should consult a holistic physician and any pertinent specialists before starting your detox program.

A short word on Supplements that augment cleansing

As earlier stated there are several brands of detox supplements on the market to augment cleansing. It is important that if you want to go on a detox program that you consult an integrative medical doctor or naturopath for the most appropriate supplements to take in your specific case. However a few supplements that are universal to cleansing are a potent multi-vitamin (remember building is a component of cleansing), a high ORAC value antioxidant of some sort (some of these will be discussed in the next chapter), a fiber supplement, and a Probiotic. I highly recommend a Superfood green as part of my cleanse, but each practitioner is different. In the next chapter, I will detail supplements that I feel are essential to have in your pantry to take on a regular basis.

3

Supplements: The Essentials

The most common question that my patients ask me is what are some essential supplements that a person should take to maintain their health. I have put together a list of supplements that would benefit anyone if taken daily.

High Potency Multivitamin. Even if you are getting the proper amount of servings of fruits, vegetables, protein and fiber, you should still take a daily multivitamin. The soil that foods are grown in today are not as nutrient rich as they used to be and vitamin and mineral deficiencies are much more prevalent today. The best vitamins to get are liquid because they are more bioavailable and more easily absorbed. I personally like the Buried Treasure VM-100 Complete, but there are many potent liquid vitamins that are of quality out there.

Superfood Greens _ SuperGreen supplements such as wheatgrass, barley grass, spirulina, or chlorella are blood building and are great sources of antioxidants. Below, I'll go over each individually, however generally they are known to lower blood pressure, cholesterol, increase the immune response, and they are anti-inflammatory in nature. There are several combination green food powders available the include the combination of these superfoods, but I particularly like Green Vibrance by Vibrant Health. Not only is it a pure and potent source of greens, but it also has many other ingredients such as omegas, probiotics, antioxidants, and adaptagens that will be covered in this chapter.

Wheatgrass

Wheatgrass is superfood that comes from the common wheat plant and is sold as either a whole juice or powder concentrate. It is typically freeze-dried if bought commercially so that it retains it's nutritional value and healing properties. It contains amino acids, proteins and enzymes. Wheatgrass is detoxifying, and to some, the wheatgrass can cause nausea with high doses of the wheatgrass. However, the benefits of wheatgrass are numerous including increased blood flow, decreased inflammation, and detoxification. It stabilizes blood sugars, helps arrest the growth of unfriendly bacteria, and normalizes bowel funtion. In an NIH study, it was shown that wheatgrass reduced the need for blood transfusions in thalassemia. In another study, wheatgrass was shown to reduce rectal bleeding and inflammation in Ulcerative Colitis patients. Wheatgrass contains chlorophyll which has been shown to lower colon cancer rates. IN breast cancer patients, a study showed the reduced need for blood and bone marrow building medications during chemotherapy. All of this suggests that the chlorophyll in wheatgrass has very powerful properties when taken regularly either in fresh juiced or powder form.

Barley Grass

Similar to wheatgrass, barley grass contains chlorophyll and abundance of vitamins, antioxidants and enzymes. In addition, barley grass has buffer minerals such as sodium, potassium, calcium and magnesium which help maintain cell integrity. Barley grass comes from the barley plant and has distinctly different properties from the barley grain. Barley grass is also known for lowering blood pressure and cholesterol. It typically is combined with wheatgrass in superfood green powder preparations, but can be purchased alone as well. Barley grass tends to be less potent and therefore doesn't have the tendency to bring on the dose related nausea that wheatgrass does.

Alfalfa grass

Alfalfa grass, again is similar to wheatgrass and barley grass. It is anti-inflammatory in nature and lowers blood pressure and cholesterol. People who have Lupus and other autoimmune disorders should not take alfalfa as it can actually flare this particular condition.

Chlorella, Spirulina and other Blue Green Algae

Chlorella, Spirulina and other blue green algae are single celled organisms that grow in fresh water. In general blue green algae improves immunity, has blood building properties, and restores good bacteria in the GI tract. Spirulina is a good vegetable source of protein as it contains the essential amino acids which are the building blocks of protein. Chlorella is a powerful deodorizer, detoxifier, and antimicrobial. It has been used in Japan to treat Peptic ulcer disease, gastritis and hypertension. It has also been used to prevent infections and protect the body from free radical damage as a result of radiation treatment in cancer patients. Chlorella, like spirulina contains 60% protein, 18 amino acids and various vitamins and minerals. Chlorella, spirulina and other blue green algaes can be bought separately but work best when combined with the superfood cereal grasses mentioned above.

Omega supplements – In addition to decreasing inflammation in the body, omega supplements are great for mood stability and brain development. Most people take fish oils, and there are many combinations. Below are some options for omegas based on your preference.

Vegetarian Omegas - Flaxseed Oil, Borage Seed Oil, Evening Primrose Oil are great options for Omega 3-6-9's if you are a vegan or vegetarian. EFA-Health from the Sun is a brand that combines all three of these. An added benefit to this vegetarian blend is that the Evening Primrose Oil is helpful for women with menopausal symptoms.

Fish Oil

Krill Oil - Krill Oil comes from a shrimp appearing crustacean in the deep seas of the far east. The oil is generally purified and cold press processed into capsuled supplemnts. Krill Oil is stud-ied to reduce inflammation in arthritis, lower LDL and triglycerides moreso then traditional fish oils. As with all fish oils, the concern for mercury content must be considered. The most important thing is to research the company reputation and check with your physician and even local whole food grocers for the best quality control brands.

Probiotics and Prebiotics – With all of the antibiotics that doctors are prescribing (not to mention the antibiotics in the meats that people eat), probiotics are necessary to prevent leaky gut syndrome from overgrowth of yeast or "bad bacteria" in our bodies. There are many combinations, but the product that I mentioned early Green Vibrance has plenty of pre – and probiotics.

Co-enzyme Q 10 – For those who have a family history or a personal history of hypertension, diabetes, heart disease of any kind, 100mg of Co-enzyme Q-10 (preferably with ALA or Alpha Lipoic Acid) is a very important addition to the supplement regimen to protect the heart and blood vessels. It has been shown to reduce the risk of heart disease and complications, and even Cardiologist are getting on board with it as a viable supplement.

Calcium & Vitamin D – Of course, for women, calcium and vitamin D are very important to protect the bones and prevent osteoporosis. However, studies are now showing that deficiency in Vitamin D may have a role in increased risk for heart disease. We are finding more and more Vitamin D deficiency today, due to the fact that we are much more inside creatures than in the old days. We work in cubicles in high rises. We tint car windows and wear SPF 50 (which is necessary to prevent skin damage and cancer), but since sun exposure is the main way that our skin activates Vitamin D production, it has become a bit of a vicious cycle that has led to deficiency. Therefore, it is essential to get it checked at your regular visits and if low, supplement with 1000mg daily until your levels are within normal.

Chia Seeds

Chia seeds are tiny seeds of the chia plant (remember the "chia pet"?). They resemble sesame seeds, and are a great source of omega 3 and fiber. Chia seeds can be eaten whole or ground and are virtually tasteless, and as such can be added to many foods including oatmeal (or any hot cereal), smoothies, salads, or even just water (if ground).

Coconut Oil

Coconut is a fruit that has been shown in research to have many healing properties. It's oil contains saturated fatty acids called medium chain triglycerides whose main components are caprylic acid and lauric acid. While previously thought to be bad for you because of it's high concentration of saturated fats, recent studies conducted on the benefits of MCT's have shown very different results. These MCT's have been shown to stablilize blood sugar, fight cancer, decrease risk for heart disease, and cure inflammation from skin diseases such as eczema or psoriasis. Coconut oil is anti-inflammatory, anti-microbial and immune boosting. In fact, a recent study showed effectiveness in the co-management of community acquired pneumonia in children. It is great for autoimmune conditions like lupus or inflammatory based conditions like Fibromyalgia. Coconut oil has been used to heal ulcers, and fight candidiasis as well as parasites. The most intriguing and promising studies today are in HIV and cancer. It is being shown that coconut oil may play a role in fighting HIV infections. Coconut oil can be bought in the raw solid oil form or in prepared capsule form. It can also be applied topically to the skin and hair (in cases of dandruff or just to maintain healthy hair). Consider either cooking with or taking coconut oil on a regular basis to decrease your overall risk for several diseases, but especially if you suffer from chronic diseases.

Meal Planning for Success

A key component to making diet transition sustainable for the long term is meal planning. This is a step that most people skip simply due to lack of awareness. With our society being as busy as it is today, it is easy for one to wake up in the morning, run out of the house and grab something on the go…. Stop for lunch at whatever convenient restaurant is near work (or worse, skip lunch), and then come home in the evening and be at the mercy of whatever happens to be in the pantry for dinner. Sound familiar? If we take just 15-20 minutes once a week, we could make eating much more organized, healthy , and less stressful. Even if you don't cook, meal planning still applies. Looking ahead allows you to be prepared for potential temptations and weak spots in your day where eating and snacking are concerned. Let's look at an example of how meal planning may help make a roller coaster eating regimen more manageable:

35

First lets look at a single corporate executive:

Jennifer is a busy corporate executive that works ten hours a day. She commutes an hour a day to work, and therefore leaves her house at 7am and gets home each day after 7pm. Jennifer used to love cooking, but lately she just doesn't have time. She generally goes out for lunch and orders in for dinner at the office when she's working late. She does make time to exercise 5 times a week, generally in the mornings before work. Her mother has diabetes, and since her father recently suffered a mild heart attack, Jennifer has become more conscious of her eating habits but is struggling to make changes due to her chaotic schedule.

Let's take another example of a busy family whose chaotic life leads to a very unhealthy eating habits that could lead to long term health consequences:

David and Laura Smith have 3 children, Danny and Kristie (ages 5 and 10, and 14), and are both full time professionals. Their children are active in dance and sports, and they seem to never have time to sit down at the table as a family for meals because of their hectic schedules. Laura gets home with the children around 7:30pm, and David gets home most days between 6pm and 7pm. Their typical family dinner is fast food that they pick up on the way home because by the time Laura gets off of work and picks up the kids she is too tired to think about cooking. David gets home and after a high pressured day takes the hour before the family gets home to unwind. Laura usually picks up something for David on the fast food stop and when everyone is home they run to their respective caves to eat, do homework and get ready for bed. Laura and David both know that their eating habits are atrocious and are no model for their children, but they are at a loss for how to change things with their unmanageable schedule.

In both of these examples, simply organizing a meal planning strategy drastically increased the likelihood that each person would be able to stick to the healthy eating regimen that they desire to create. It is important to know that meal planning doesn't always involve cooking. It simply means that you have formulated a plan of action for how you are going to manage your diet for the planning time period, be it a week, a month, or just for the day. Below are 10 simple steps to organizing an eating plan that will fit your lifestyle needs.

1. *Recognize whether you are a cook or not.*

It is very important to recognize and acknowledge first of all whether you like to cook and also whether you are good at it.

If you feel you are not good at cooking, the next thing to figure out is if you are willing to better your skills by learning simple recipes and building over time. If you are a good cook, or are willing to improve your skills, then the next step is applicable. If you are not a cook and don't have a desire to learn, or if you just do not like to cook, you will want to find a number of healthy restaurants, café's, or deli's from which you can make healthy selections. Alternatively, you may choose to hire a personal chef to pre-prepare meals for your week, buy prepared healthy meals and have them delivered, or purchase prepared healthy frozen meals to eat instead. The first two options are a bit more pricey, but are the better choice for freshness and taste, and are probably more nutritious in the long run. However if you are on a budget, frozen meals are not a bad option so long as you read the labels and make healthy choices.

2. *Define your specific tastes*
Knowing what you like will make it easier for your to design a meal plan that has some variety. Think about what you definitely like, what you have always been curious about trying, and explore new tastes that you may not have even considered. Healthy eating doesn't have to be bland. In fact, it can be quite exciting.

3. Identify the challenges in your schedule

This is probably the most crucial. If you can identify the challenges in your schedule, you can begin to troubleshoot solutions. In the case of the corporate executive, she worked late hours and has a long commute. She may choose to cook on Sundays for dinner, and pre-prepare her lunches at night before she goes to bed or order in from a healthy restaurant for lunch. In the case of the chaotic family, between Laura's, the kids', and David's schedules, they just couldn't coordinate meal preparation. Knowing this she can brainstorm several solutions for shopping and preparing meals during the week.

4. Pick a day of the week to make a plan for your eating for the week

If you pick a day of the week to make a plan for your next week's eating, it will make creating your shopping list much easier (which will in turn, make your shopping much more efficient and easy).

5. Make a shopping list according to that plan

This is pretty self explanatory. Making a shopping list according to what you are going to prepare for the week will ensure that you don't overspend, that you won't get off track and buy things you don't need, and that you won't overshop and end up wasting food in the end.

6. *If cooking pick 1, 2, or 3 days that you will prepare the meals according to your schedule and convenience*

It often takes come of the pressure off having to cook daily if you pre-prepare your meals on one or two days of the week for the remainder of the week. You can either store the food in large or individual containers. Some even prepare the food and freeze them for warming the day of to keep the relative freshness. Either way, cooking or pre-preparing your meals is just another way to make keeping a healthy diet a little more sustainable and manageable.

7. If there is a spouse or family involved, engage them for help in the planning in order to further make the process more manageable.

For many families, one person bears the burden of food preparation, shopping, and cooking. This does not have to be the case. Even if only one spouse can cook in the home, the other can provide simple help such as chopping vegetables or warming food in the evenings if it's pre-cooked. Also, spouses can work together on lunch preparations the night before if they have early schedules. They may take turns to keep the burden from being with one person. In addition, engaging the spouse can actually bring pleasure or even romance to the cooking activity. Engaging the children can make prepration fun for the children while at the same time modeling healthy behavior. Giving the children something simple to do like stirring or mixing a ingredients, helping add spices or herbs to the dish, or even putting measured food into the cooking pot. Of course, if your children are helping you cook, close supervision is required to keep them safe. But, consider making cooking a family affair. It could be another way to make the family bond stronger. The same applies to romantic or spousal relationships.

8. *Account for deviations from the plan. Have a backup plan in place.*

We all know that there will always be deviations from the normal schedule sometimes. "Stuff happens". The key is what we do when things get off track. For example, if you travel out of town and therefore are not able to do your normal shopping and cooking regimen, you might identify healthy restaurants to pick up food instead. If you know you will be traveling away from your home, you might prepare a meal and freeze it so you don't have to worry about meal planning the week you get back. There are many ways to remain one step ahead of the game so that you can maintain control of your diet. If you have a back up plan, then you are less likely to be thrown off track when plans go awry.

9. *Consider having an accountability partner if you know you have trouble sticking to plans*

Sticking to a new plan can be challenging, and there are many temptations that catch the eye designed to lead us astray. If you are one that has a tendency to fall to the temptation, consider having an accountability partner. If you are a family, you can keep each other accountable. If you are a single, find a friend that you can call when things get tough and you feel like taking the easy unhealthy road. You can even engage your work colleagues or your neighborhood. The more people involved the more fun it can become, and the more likely your success. Don't underestimate the power of peer encouragement.

10. *Stick to the plan*

Well, this is self explanatory. Remember that at first the transition will be challenging. You will need to work out the kinks as you go along to fit your own style of living. It takes

21 days to form a habit. This is one that is well worth the work. Once you have gotten the routine down, it will be like second nature, and a healthy life will be much more manageable than you may have imagined.

Now, to show you what these steps might look like altogether, I've taken the Smith family and created one solution for their chaotic dietary habits. Let's say Laura makes her shopping list on Fridays, shops on Saturdays, and prepares two meals for the week for dinner on Sundays. She can engage her 10 and 14 year old for help on the Sunday preparation, and engage the husband's help to warm the food for dinner during the week. In addition, on Sundays she might engage to family to help prepare snacks to carry along in the car for eating between after school activities and arriving home. See how applying these simple steps creates a routine that has the family working together and takes the pressure off of any one spouse for total responsibility for meal management?

Now it's your turn. Take some time and apply these steps to your situation. Write about how these steps may fit into your lifestyle and make things more manageable for you. Then put that written plan into action. Now, we move on to the next step: Shopping.

EAT YOUR DISEASE AWAY

5

Healthy Shopping Made Practical

What's in your kitchen? Don't you just love when you go to the doctor and the doctor says, "Well, you need to eat a healthier diet." And you're wondering – well yeah, I know that, but how exactly do I start? Well, that's what we're about to talk about. Getting your nutrition on track starts the minute you walk into your local grocery store or farmer's market. In this chapter we're going to learn how to identify unhealthy foods in your cabinet, understand why they're considered unhealthy, learn why labels are important, and learn how to read them, create a healthy shopping list, and then learn great tips on when, where, and how to shop effectively.

So what's in your cabinet? Do you have canned foods, pasta, white rice, bleached flour or white sugar? Do you have taco mix, canned soup, or powdered soup mix? Do you have MSG-containing products, sugar cereals? Or do you have dried herbs and spices, sugar substitutes, herbal teas? Maybe you have raw or turbinado sugar, unbleached wheat or spelt flour, organic broths, soups, or carton soups. Perhaps you have whole grains such as quinoa, oats, and high-fibre breakfast cereal.

What's in your refrigerator? Maybe you have whole milk, cheeses, non-organic fruit juices or canned fruit. Perhaps you have diet sodas, butters, beer, or wine. Or maybe you have low fat skimmed milk or milk alternatives such as almond or soy milk, low fat cheeses, fresh fruit, fresh vegetables, fresh herbs, margarines, or free-range eggs.

What's in your freezer? Frozen pizzas? Frozen TV dinners? Ice creams? Frozen family sized meals? Perhaps you have frozen meats such as red meat, chicken, or pork. Maybe you have organic meats such as chicken or low-mercury fish. Perhaps you have frozen vegetables or frozen juice concentrates.

Any of these sound familiar? Why is it even important? Largely because it's essential to know what you already have before you can change it.

Try this exercise. Take an inventory of your pantry, of your refrigerator, of your spice cabinet, and then your freezer.

Now that you have inventoried your kitchen, how do you make your shopping list? Do you make it according to what you think you need, or do you make it according to what you're about to cook for the week?

Here's another exercise: make yourself a sample shopping list for the coming week. What does your shopping list look like? Is it balanced? Does it include a variety of grains, fruits and vegetables? Or does it include the things that you just think you need for the week?

In this chapter we will be discussing efficient shopping and a bit more meal planning, but for now let's move on to what the contents of the shopping list should look like.

Going shopping

Canned vs frozen vs fresh

Let's talk first about canned, fresh, and frozen. What's the big deal about canned fruits and vegetables? Why are they considered less healthy than the others? Well, typically canned fruits and vegetables are often thought of as less fresh, but actually, the studies are inconsistent. It's thought that the processing destroys the vitamins and mineral content, and you have a significant loss in fibre. Lots of times canned vegetables are overcooked, thereby having a less nutritional value and canned fruits are soaked in sugary syrups that contain high fructose corn syrup and are clearly detrimental to our health. In addition, many canned vegetables have an added preservative or salt content to them as well and canned fruits have an additional sugar added as well. However, there are canned fruits and vegetables that have no preservatives, no sugar added, no salt added, and are considered organic. So then, what is the main difference between fresh and canned fruits and vegetables? It's the taste. Fruits and veggies that are fresh are best when eaten soon after picked, but over time even, some of the vitamins and minerals in fresh fruits and vegetables, if left out, are subject to oxidation with time and therefore the nutritional content goes down. However, choosing fresh fruits and fresh vegetables as opposed to canned gives you a wider variety of choices in your meals.

What about frozen? Well, frozen is a better choice when it comes to frozen or canned. Generally, frozen vegetables or fruit are flash frozen just after the harvest, so they retain their nutritional value. Usually with frozen fruits or vegetables, no preservatives, salts, and sugars are added, so they are a good alternative to fresh produce. But, of course, nothing beats the taste of fresh fruits and vegetables.

Organic vs nonorganic

Okay, so now let's talk about organic versus non-organic. What's the big difference? Well, typically our non-organic vegetables and fruits contain many pesticides which can cause cancer and other illness. The non-organic meats typically contain hormones and antibiotics which we ingest when we eat the meat. When you eat meat that has its own hormones, it can add – especially for women, but even in men – can add hormones to our own bodies that we don't need, and that in itself can cause disease.

Non-organic vegetables and fruits are not eco friendly and typically, because of the soil that they're grown in, are not as high in nutritional value. This is because the soil is turned and reused and the pesticides seep into the soil so that the vegetables contain less of a nutritional content than the ones that are organically grown. Also, non-organic fruits and vegetables expose farmers to pesticides. However, sometimes it's difficult to buy organic all the time, and even sometimes – the way our society is – more expensive. So if you're buying non-organic fruits and vegetables, be sure to wash them with a veggie wash before ingesting them.

If shopping organic, you'll find that organic fruits and vegetables have a much richer taste and they actually even look brighter. Your strawberries are redder; your apples are crisper, than your non-organic fruits and vegetables. When shopping organic, you want to look for signs that say "USDA Organic, Non-GMO" That means there's no genetic modification. In addition, if you're shopping for organic meats, you want to make sure the animals are grass-fed, free-range, and are not infused with hormones or antibiotics.

Microwaving

Moving on, let's talk about microwavables. Microwaving is convenient, but at what cost? Microwaving alters the natural food structures of our food or beverage. It kills the vitamins and minerals and the toxins from the microwavable containers can leak into the food. Alternatives to microwaving include warming on the stovetop, using convection ovens, toaster ovens, and conventional oven warming. Let's think about the microwave in our home and every time we turn on the microwave, how we're exposing ourselves to radiation. Sure, people may say, that is minimal radiation coming from that microwave. But if you think about us using that microwave every day for 20 or 30 years, that's a significant exposure to radiation. If you compound that on our exposure to cell phones, Bluetooth, computers, and other types of radiation, having a microwave to cook our food is just adding to the process of inflammation and cellular dysfunction in our body.

I'll share with you a quick way that my aunt taught me how to warm my food. My aunt lives in New York and she doesn't own a microwave. Once I went up to visit her and she had a pot of boiling water on which she set a bowl of cold soup. She then put the top over the cold soup and allowed the steam from the boiling water to rise up and warm up the soup. It took just as much time as one minute in the microwave and tasted great. I soon adopted this technique and have improvised upon it. I have a large pot with a steam basket and now, what I do, is I take a small plate with my food, and I place my food in the steam basket, putting the top on top of the pot and allowing the steam to quickly warm the entire plate. It takes less than five minutes and the food tastes delicious.

The other method I like to use is I place my plate or I place a casserole dish with my food in it in the oven and cover it with foil. Then I turn the broiler on. This warms the oven up faster and from the top and allows the food to be warmed without being dried or burned. You can also, if you're warming in a casserole dish, place just a little bit of water in the casserole dish so the food stays moist and creates a steam within the pot that you're warming up. I encourage you to try some of these alternative methods of rewarming food and soon you may find that you're disposing of your own microwave.

Dairy and Fats

Let's continue our shopping sprees. On to dairy and fats. Dairy contains calcium and other nutrients, so it is important to

get your dairy in. However, buying organic avoids the hormones and the antibiotics that the dairy products may contain as
they do come from the same cows that we're trying to avoid
with all those antibiotics and hormones.

Free range eggs are preferable to traditional eggs, and if
you're lactose intolerant there are several alternatives to milk
including rice, almond, and hemp. Soy milk is also an alternative but you need to be careful because many of the soy products
these days are genetically modified. In addition, too much soy
has been linked to some thyroid diseases and, because of the estrogen content of soy, it's important that if you're a breast cancer
patient or survivor and especially if you are estrogen receptor
positive, it's important that you do not take in soy products because they are a natural source of estrogen and you want to
avoid this in your case.

On to fats and butters. Generally, it's a good idea to avoid
your lards and your solid butters if possible. However, there is a
type of clarified butter called 'ghee' that has healing properties
in irovetic medicine. So go ahead and look for the ghee and that
has a butter taste – you can use that as a spread and in cooking,
if needed. Margarine, in particular, is found to have no real nutritional value and often is genetically modified. The best oils to
use are extra virgin olive oil, sunflower oil, and canola in cooking.

Beverages

Continuing our shopping spree on to beverages, let's talk about the beverages that should be limited or avoided. Generally, the thing to avoid in beverages is your black coffees, your black tea, and your sodas or carbonated drinks. Juices that should be avoided are your non-organic juices such as Tang, Sunny D, apple juices, Kool-Aid and the likes of drinks. Now if I've just eliminated everything in your pantry, don't cry! There are plenty of beverages to enjoy; you just have to be a little open to trying new things. Go for organic juices – orange, apple, cranberry and the likes. There are plenty of 100% juices out there. Just make sure you look at the labels and that that 100% juice isn't from some sugary concentrate.

Water is a great beverage. Some people hate the taste of water, so what I encourage them to do is get a little Crystal Lite. Crystal Lite in water will give it some taste, and you will still be able to have great hydration value. For the people who are caffeine lovers, green teas and black herbal teas such as orange pekoe or Chinese white tea are good alternatives to your black coffees. However, if you want to drink coffee – if you just love the taste coffee – then try to limit your coffee to one cup a day.

Other great beverages to enjoy are smoothies, which can actually be a meal substitute, almond milk, which is rich and tastes the close to real milk as I've experienced, and if you must have your traditional milk, just go for the 2% or low fat milk. And, of course, remember to choose organic, as we've said previously in this book.

Sweeteners

We're on to sweeteners. If you're anything like me, this is the most important food group of them all: sugar. Typically you want to avoid your refined white sugars. I have worked very hard in my lifetime to replace what I grew up with – which was the classic Dominos, dark brown sugar, or the regular white sugar – but what I've found over the years is that I've been introduced to a number of substitutes to those unhealthy refined sugars that taste great.

First of all, turbinado or sugar in the raw, or is a lot less refined than your traditional white sugar. However, it's still sugar and you want to avoid too much of any sugar, because it can lead to overgrowth of yeast and Candida in the body. It also leads to obesity and diabetes as well as chronic fatigue.

Other healthy substitutes for sugar include Zylitol. Zylitol is a type of sugar that's actually found in toothpaste. It's considered one of the healthy sugars because it actually helps decrease decay of the teeth.

Sweeteners outside of the sugar family that can be enjoyed are things like stevia and agave nectar. Agave nectar is one of my favorite sweeteners. It appears like honey, but with the consistency of syrup, and it tastes as sweet as the real thing. It's not too sweet and it doesn't have an aftertaste. I use agave nectar in my teas, to sweeten my cereals, my oatmeals, and in any other dish that I might normally use my traditional brown sugar or white sugar.

I also love stevia. Stevia has been a controversial one for most of the people that I know because they say that it has an aftertaste. But the key to using stevia is if you use it to enhance the natural sweetness of your natural sugars, such as turbinado or agave nectar. You can use stevia in your tea, in your coffee, in place of things like splenda or aspartame (which is commonly known as Equal). Since Equal has been linked to migraines and cancer, it's best that you avoid it at all cost. In addition, you really want to avoid your Sweet-n-Lows, which is saccharine, because that also has been linked to cancers in laboratory animals.

Splenda has even now been found to be harmful. Do you know what Splenda is? Splenda is a chlorinated sugar. That means someone took a regular sugar molecule and put some chlorine with it, and voila, you have Splenda. How can that possibly be healthy for you? In addition, Splenda has been linked to problems with the thyroid and has been linked to cancer in laboratory animals. What's more, since Splenda is a relatively new sweetener, there are not many long-term studies on it, so who knows what kind of problems could come forth later on from this chlorinated sugar.

So, to review, use stevia, agave nectar, SlimSweet, Zylitol, or turbinado sugar and even raw honey in place of refined, white sugars, molasses, NutriSweet, aspartame, Splenda, and Sweet-n-Low.

Carbs and grains

All right, we're moving right on through the grocery store. Let's continue on to our carbs and fibre. When we break down grains, carbs, and fibers, we're breaking them down into good carbs versus bad carbs. The good carbs tend to be low to medium glycemic index, which means they don't cause major highs and lows of the insulin and blood sugar in the body. These low to medium glycemic index grains include:

Whole grain pastas
Whole grain bread
Wild or brown rice
Quinoa
Millet
Legumes
Lentils, beans and peas

Let's talk a little bit about the grain quinoa. It's one of my favorite grains to cook. Basically, if you're familiar with cous-cous, quinoa appears like couscous or a small ball of rice, except for it has a small sprout on the end. The great thing about quinoa is that it's wholesome in flavor, but it's also a great high source of protein and fiber. Quinoa can be used in place of any rice, millet, or couscous; it can be eaten with gravies or even made as a cereal. Later on in this series we're going to talk about how to utilize your grains such as cous cous and quinoa, and how to utilize you legumes such as lentils, beans, and peas to create great, wholesome, and anti—inflammatory recipes.

Meat

Onward to our meat choices. For those who are not vegetarian, it is important to know what meat choices are healthiest and what meats are the cleanest. In general, red meat is not easily digested and usually contains hormones and antibiotics. This makes it not the most efficient meat for your digestive process and it can block absorption and build up in the colon, causing leaky gut syndrome. Pork usually contains high sodium content and fat content. Typically, the animals that are pork animals are scavengers, so if you can imagine eating what a scavenger eats, then you can imagine what you're eating when you're eating pork.

Poultry, if not free range, can also contain hormones. Seafood, while usually healthy, can contain high mercury levels in some types. So what are your healthiest, cleanest red meats to partake? Typically deer meat (also known as venison), goat meat, lamb, and calf or veal are your cleanest red meats to partake. They don't contain as many hormones or antibiotics and they're usually grass fed or free range.

In terms of chicken, you want to make sure you look at the label for grass fed, free range, or no hormones and antibiotics injected. This is the chicken you want to choose. You'll taste the difference in both your red meats and your chicken and poultry if you buy them clean, meaning without genetic modification, without hormones, without pesticides, and without antibiotics.

Now let's talk a little bit about fish. Fish are generally healthy, but you must beware of two things: the mercury content and the preparation method in the grocery stores. Let's address the mercury content first. High mercury fish include shark, swordfish, ahi tuna, yellowfin tuna, sea bass, and some blue fish groupers. These are the mercury-containing fish that you want to avoid. Moderate mercury-containing fish should be limited to less than six servings per month. Some examples of these are Atlantic halibut, skip shack tuna, snapper, skate, perch, stripped and black bass, and Alaskan carp cod. Some of these fishes I never eat anyway, so that's not a problem.

The fish with the least amount of mercury are the fish that you can enjoy the most – and there are plenty of these. Some of these include your domestic crab, your croaker, flounder, herring, North Atlantic mackerel, salmon (canned or fresh), your scallops, shrimp, calamari (or squid), tilapia, trout, white fish, and whiting. So as you can see, there are plenty of low mercury containing fish that you can enjoy.

The great thing about fish, especially salmon, is that they contain omega acids and that's very good for anti-inflammation and for the heart.

The second thing to address with fish is the cleaning practices. Be cautious when you buy the fish at the grocery store, because some fish in regular supermarkets are washed with chlorine based, toxic washes. Just like you don't want to be eating a chlorinate sugar, you don't want to be eating a chlorinated fish. So go to your local farmer's market, where the fish are fresh.

We've covered all the food groups and now there's just one more thing to address: snacks. Of course we're going to be cooking some, we're going to be choosing food in restaurants, but oftentimes during the day we like to snack – or at least I know I do. So let's go over what the difference between healthy snacks and non-healthy snacks are.

Better yet, let's have a little *pop quiz*.

True or false: the following snacks are healthy.

Potato chips?

Beef or turkey jerky ?

Pringles?

Pretzels?

Popcorn?

Snickers?

Oatmeal cookies?

Cheezits?

What about baked rice chips or ginger snaps?

Soy beans, also called edamame?

Sunflower or pumpkin seeds?

Strawberries?

Apples?

My guess is you have the right answers to which snacks are healthy and which snacks are not. So when you shop, think about your snacks. Think about what you want to choose that's healthy before you go into the grocery store, so you don't just gravitate to the potato chip section and then pick up those Pringles because, hey, they're right in front of me and I know I'm going to be needing some snacks sometime. Doesn't work like that. Later on in this series, when we talk more specifically about healthy cooking and also – in a bonus segment of this book called Six Small Meals – we will explore quick tips and tricks to choosing and even making your own healthy snacks.

Okay, we've covered a lot of ground in this healthy shopping chapter, but there's just one more thing to do. That thing is to recreate your shopping list! At the end of this chapter, make another shopping list based on what you know about what we've talked about in this chapter.

How has your shopping list changed? Compare it with your old shopping list. Share it with someone else. Do you feel like you have a handle on what should be on the shopping list? If not, that's okay. It's a process. You can refer back to this chapter as often as you'd like in order to get what you need on making your healthy shopping list.

Now let's go over a few more shopping tips to help you to optimize your grocery shopping, save money, and avoid the temptations of unhealthy buying. Let's start with traditional grocery store tips.

To avoid the temptation of the unhealthy foods, its best to shop the perimeter of the grocery store first. You'll find your produce, your meats, your frozen and your dairy are on the outside. Also, get in the habit of reading your labels. Look at fibre, grams, carbs, sugar and fat calorie content of the food. Never go shopping on an empty stomach – you're more likely to impulse shop that way and buy your sugars and your unhealthy snacks. Think twice before buying forbidden foods. Do you really need it, or are you just craving it at the moment? Resist, resist, resist! Always take a shopping list and don't deviate from it. Make your shopping list based on the meals that you're planning for the week. This helps you to avoid buying what you don't need. It also helps to avoid impulse buying. In the end, it'll also save you a lot of money. We'll talk more about meal planning later on in this chapter.

So now you know your options. What do you do now? Make a list with healthy choice. Plan your meals for the week. Make your shopping list based on the meal plans for the week, and shop only for that week if you're able. Plan healthy snacks and plan to take your lunch with you to work instead of eating out. Again, remember – if this is too much information for you to digest all at one time, you have plenty of opportunity to re-listen to this over and over again, take notes, and apply these principles to your shopping.

Next we're going to talk about healthy cooking and how to incorporate fun, easy, simple tips into your cooking for both people who love to cook and people who don't like it so much.

6

Healthy Cooking

Who said that healthy eating had to be boring or taste bland? In the last chapter on healthy shopping, we learned how healthy nutrition starts as soon as you walk into the grocery store. Well when you get home, where do you walk into to put the groceries up? The answer is your kitchen, of course! In this chapter we will discuss different ways to put recipes together using various ingredients and preparation methods.

We learned in the last chapter how to inventory our kitchen. Let's do that again now. What's currently in your pantry? Brown rice or wild rice? Do you have pasta? Soup bases like broths, oatmeals, quinoa, millet? Do you have dry beans like black beans or pinto beans, red beans, lentils? How about unbleached wheat or spelt flour? Corn meal? Almonds, nuts or seeds? Barley? Flax seeds? Do you have packaged or canned salmon tuna? What about granola? These may seem random but all of them are components that can make great meals.

What about your refrigerator? Do you have low fat or skimmed milk or milk alternatives? Do you have low fat cheeses, fresh fruits like lemons, limes, oranges, bananas or strawberries? What about fresh vegetables? Do you have legumes such a squash, eggplant or potatoes? What about margarines or butters? Ghee, as we talked about in the last chapter? Do you have red wine or marinades? Free range eggs? Fresh herbs or spices such as cilantro, chives, onion, parsley, and dill? What's in your freezer? Organic bread and meats? Organic chickens? Low mercury fish? Frozen vegetables? Frozen fruits? Frozen juice concentrates? Tofu, tempeh, or Seitan? And what's in your spice cabinet? Do you have any thyme, marjoram, basil, dried cilantro and chives? Do you have pepper, cinnamon, and allspice? What about lemon pepper, curry powder, turmeric, organic chili powder? Do you have any mixed seasonings such as chipotle or masalas? The reason we are inventorying this time is not for the health purposes so much as to know what are the different varieties of things that you have in your refrigerator to provide a variety of great tasting and healthy meals. All the things aforementioned are all components to make a variety of different, tasty meals. Most people prepare with butters, fats, some prepare with olive oil, salts, peppers, and season-all, like Mrs. Dash or seasoned salts. While these are good, there are so many things out there that can add variety to your cooking. Take herbs and spices, for example. How many people that you know regularly use herbs and spices in their cooking? Herbs and spices like garlic, oregano, cilantro, onion, lemon and lime zest, dill and dill weed, cumin, turmeric, saffron, sage, basil, marjoram, ginger, cinnamon, nutmeg, parsley, fennel, coriander, curry, chives, bay, and horseradish. If it seems that I'm slightly excited by these, it's because I've used all of these in my cooking and I can't tell you what a difference it makes for me to have the variety of using all of these different spices so that I don't get bored in my cooking and in my eating. It's important to know that the herbs and spices not only make your food taste good, but many of them actually have health benefits as well and I want to go over a few of these health benefits to impress upon you that anti-inflammatory eating actually includes the use of herbs and spices.

Let's start with basil.

Basil has a reputation for stimulating the appetite and the nervous system. It's commonly used in the Far East in cough medicines and it relieves kidney and diarrhea problems. Well, commonly, we use basil in a lot of our Italian food. Take some

65

time to sprinkle basil over a soup that you make, a vegetable soup or even a chicken noodle soup.

Cinnamon. Cinnamon is a strong glandular stimulant. Some of the glands in our body include the adrenal glands and the thyroid glands. Cinnamon was given as a sedative to mothers during childbirth. It's also an antacid for helping upset stomachs and diarrhea. Years ago it was also commonly used as a breath sweetener. I love to add cinnamon to my warm cereals such as oatmeal or cream of wheat.

Clove. Clove can relieve the suffering of an aching tooth. Clove also tastes great in cereals such as oats, cream of wheat, or creamed barley. Clove has a nice and sweetly pungent smell and also is very nice in Caribbean dishes – commonly used, I believe, in jerk seasonings.

Cumin, fennel and ginger are spices commonly used in Indian cooking. Cumin seeds have been used since the Bible times and are calming in digestive problems. Fennel can be used to help digestion as well and is used to baby's cripe water. It can be used as a breath sweetener, for ear aches, toothaches, and helps relieve coughs and asthma. If you soak the seeds in water, they make a very soothing lotion for sore and tired eyes.

Ginger

In ancient India, ginger is considered to be an essential part of the diet and especially in protection of disease. Ginger has natural antiseptic properties that help with colds and sore throats. Pickled ginger is also used alongside of Sushi. I have personally found ginger to be a natural antiviral. Whenever I begin sniffling or having any type of scratchy throat or achy body, I cut a piece of ginger, boil it for 15 to 20 minutes, add a little lemon and honey, and drink it as a tea. In no time my sore throat and my achy body has gone straight away. I usually combine the ginger with 3000 milligrams of vitamin C to boost the immune system, so keep that in mind for your cold and flu season.

Horseradish has antibiotic properties that protect the colon from harmful bacteria. It also encourages circulation, clears the sinuses and is excellent for insect bites, cuts, and stings. Apparently it is also effective in eliminating acne. Horseradish has a kick to it and is typically used as a dipping sauce for things like calamari or raw vegetables.

Nutmeg goes great with hot oatmeal or cream of wheat and is medicinally used in helping with gas and vomiting.

Rosemary. It has been discovered that rosemary has been able to expand tissues, increasing blood flow, which is beneficial to the heart and the blood vessels for circulation. It is even believed to stimulate hair growth. Rosemary is also excellent sprinkled on baked chicken or fish for added flavor.

Sage has many cleansing properties and is also good for the nerves and blood. It can be applied as a wash to improve conditions of the skin and hair. Sage is also very good in vegetable soups, chicken broths, and in baked chicken, typically stuffed with potatoes.

Thyme. Because its leaves contain the volative oil thymal, this herb has been a disinfectant and can be used as a poultice. It can be mixed with honey to soothe a raw throat, or can be used as a mouthwash and natural toothpaste. Studies have also shown that thyme is a great anti-fungal, along with tea tree. I love to add thyme to many things including scrambled eggs, broccoli cream soup, cream of potato soup, cream of tomato soup (notice I like soups!). I love to add it to my baked chicken or pan fried chicken, even. It's just a great seasoning overall to add to any food preparation.

Now that we've covered just a few of the spices that can enhance any meal, let's talk about some quick preparation methods. When I do my lunch and learns for the different corporations, one of the most common things that I get is, "I don't have time to cook. I want my meals to be prepared in 30 minutes or less." Believe me, as a busy professional, I definitely can resonate with that and I am all about efficiency in cooking. So let's talk about a couple of quick food preparation methods that have worked for me as well as the audiences that I've spoken to in the past.

First is *casseroling*. Casseroling is a great preparation method because the overall packaging is easy. You have one pot, with multiple ingredients and you can easily scoop it out, put it in a Tupperware, and carry it to work the next day. Some great ideas for great ideas for casseroling are tuna casserole, broccoli and rice casserole, even Mexican-style casseroling like enchiladas and Mexican pizzas are great and easy to prepare.

Most casseroles can be prepared in 30 minutes or less including cook time and last for two to three days. Later on I'll give you some easy casseroling recipes that you can add to your database.

Steaming. Earlier we talked about steaming as a rewarming method, but steaming is a quick prep method that can be done in five minutes or less. You can steam veggies – my favorite to steam are broccoli or asparagus – or you can even steam meats, such as fish, which are very very quick, salmon, tuna, or even things like tilapia or whiting. All you have to do is put the herbs and the spices over the fish or the meat, or go ahead and sprinkle the herbs and salts or lemon over the vegetables, and steam for five to ten minutes. With meats, of course, the steaming process will be a little bit longer, but not by much.

One of the nice things about steaming is that it can be done alongside of other preparation methods, so for example, if you have a steaming pot that has a basket, you can place the water in and boil some pasta while steaming the vegetables on top. At the end of the day you can strain the pasta, place your veggies on top, maybe add a little parmesan cheese and olive oil, and you have yourself a great, easy meal in approximately 10 minutes.

Stir-frying is another 30 minute or less preparation method. If you have a taste for Asian flavor, throw some sprouts, some broccoli, some watercress, some snap peas, and maybe a little chicken into a wok – it can be an electric wok or a stovetop wok – and you can stir-fry your veggies, adding just a little bit of soy sauce or Bragg's Liquid Aminos (even better) and have a great meal in just about 20 minutes.

Pan searing, which is a very easy way to prepare meat or even the hard vegetables such as eggplant, is a very easy and quick way to create a nice meal. I like to blacken chicken or fish every now and then and put it on top of a salad. Later on I'll give you some great recipes that involve pan searing, blackening, and even pan searing with jerk seasoning.

Sautéing is another very quick, easy way to prepare your vegetables, your meats, or your seafood. I love to sauté scallops over garlic in olive oil and then add them to a whole grain pasta with a little bit of parmesan cheese on top. As you can see, one of the things I really love is Italian food. This is a quick, easy, and relatively healthy way to indulge your Italian flair.

Pressure-cooking. One of the things I like about pressure cooking is that things that normally take a little bit longer to cook, such as wild grains like wild rice or wild quinoa, and legumes such as red beans or black beans, can be made in about 30 minutes with a pressure cooker. Pressure cookers are easy to find. You can buy them at your local Wal-Mart, Target, or a local grocery store. Pressure cooking expands the amount of foods that you're able to cook in a little bit of time.

Can you think of any preparation methods that are very quick that I didn't mention? If so, write them down. Create the list.

Now we've talked a little bit about food preparation methods, here are some examples of some preparation ideas throughout the food groups. I spoke a little bit about blackened chicken and fish, sautéed scallops – what about broiled turkey, Stewed fishes in a red sauce; Casseroled chicken; and veggies which you can wok stir fry as I mentioned earlier. You can roast vegetables in the oven, which actually doesn't take that long because vegetables cook fairly quickly or you can sauté your vegetables. Finally, of course, as earlier mentioned, casseroling such as your broccoli-rice casserole is a great food preparation method. Legumes, such as potatoes can be roasted in the oven with a little rosemary on top and olive oil. You can bake your potatoes. You can actually boil and mash potatoes, particularly I like boiled and mashed yams – it indulges my sweet tooth.

Also, one easy thing to cook is beans and rice. Again, using the pressure cooker, it cuts down the time of cooking the dry bean which might take an hour to two hours to less than 30 minutes.

And then of course your grains are going to be me mostly either steamed, broiled, or sautéed, in the case of rice.

Are you seeing how, just by using a variety of preparation methods, you can increase the variety of foods that you eat? Varying your preparation methods means you don't have to get bored, nor do you have to spend an hour slaving over the stove after work.

Here are a few more preparation ideas using herbs and marinades. My friend, Wendy Battles, who is a clean eating coach, loves to zest. She loves using orange, lemon, or lime zest over many of her breakfast and dinner preparations. You can use orange or pineapple juice in addition to that as a marinade. Combining a fresh apple juice, pineapple juice, an apple cider or balsamic vinaigrette and olive oil also makes a great salad dressing.

If you like international foods, don't forget about things like jerk seasoning. Not only does jerk go well with your meats such as chicken, shrimp or other seafood, but it can go very well on vegetables such as eggplant.

Curry is a great way to infuse Indian or Caribbean flavor into any of your means. I love to do curry lentils and wrap them in a whole grain tortilla.

You can add thyme, basil, marjoram, and sea salt to a red wine or a white vinegar wine if you're making cream sauce, to create a very nice marinade or to create a very nice sauté sauce for a pasta or meat.

Dill weed, thyme, and white wine vinegar can be added to mushroom soup for a great chicken, beef, or scallop sauce.

And also, using Bragg's Liquid Aminos as I earlier mentioned can add a soy sauce like flavor to your stir fried vegetables.

I want you to keep in mind that, as I go through these healthy cooking meal ideas, I'm using mostly foods from the alkaline group. As we reviewed earlier, alkaline decreases inflammation in the body and the whole purpose of switching to a more nutritious and healthy diet is so that we can decrease the inflammation in the body, thereby halting or reversing disease processes that may be going on in our body. And for those of us who are healthy, we maintain our healthy status and continue our quality of life as it is.

I want to move on to using legumes. Let's talk about the different varieties of legumes that there are. Many people are very familiar with red beans, black beans, and pinto beans, but not so many are as familiar with lentils, chickpeas, garbanzos, mung beans, and aduke beans. These are all alkaline producing beans that can be prepared all in the same way by boiling and put over rice, curried, put in a red sauce stew, made into chilies, or any other type of variety of preparation that you have a taste for. The beans that are easiest to cook are chickpeas and lentils. These two peas can be cooked within a 20-minute period. One of the things that I like to do with chickpeas which may seem odd is to boil them and actually mash them. If you mash chickpeas and add a little salt and pepper and thyme, it actually tastes like mashed potatoes – except it's got a higher protein value and it'll stick to you a little bit longer. It's also low-glycemic in nature so it doesn't cause those fluctuations in insulin and sugar that we talked about earlier.

While mung beans and aduke beans seem like a strange bean, they can be prepared just like the black bean, the red bean, or the pinto bean.

Let's look at our potato family. There are different varieties of potatoes including your regular, white Idaho potatoes, your red potatoes, your creamer potatoes, sweet potatoes, yams, and eucham. The thing about white Idaho potatoes is that these days there are a lot of them that are genetically modified, so you really have to be careful about those. The red potatoes actually have a richer taste and the skin can be easier eating. I like to frequently use red potatoes instead of white potatoes, especially in my leek cream of potato soup, which I'll give you the recipe for later on in the book.

Another thing that I really love to do is mash sweet potatoes and yams. I may have mentioned this earlier, but for me and for others who may have a sweet tooth, sweet potatoes are a great nutritional source and they also curb the sweet craving. Yams do the same thing and if you're into, again, a variety of types of potatoes, or potato-like foods, you ought to try to euchum, which is generally from Central American and the Caribbean and has a sweet taste to itself. You just peel it, boil it, and mash it up.

I know this is a lot of information, but we're at the ninth inning here so stay with me and let's get on with great grains for variety.

We've talked about – in the inflammatory diet – how refined foods contribute to inflammation at the cellular level. So some of the grains that are great anti-inflammatory grains are wild rice and brown rice, quinoa, cous cous, amaranth, and millet. I know I'm introducing some new names to you, and I know also that the things like wild rice and brown rice typically take a little bit longer to cook, but if you remember we talked about pressure cooking and how pressure cooking can cut down on the time for those traditional wild and brown rice type of grains that take longer to cook to less than 30 or 20 minutes.

Let's talk a little bit more about *quinoa*, which I described earlier as a small grain that's very similar to the couscous grain except for it has a little sprout on the end. Quinoa comes in a traditional variety or a red and wild variety. It can be eaten as a breakfast cereal or alongside a major meal, like rice. It's great mixed with gravies and sauces, and it's a low-glycemic, high-protein, and has a wholesome taste. Really give thought to this grain as it has some of the best properties of all of the following listed grains with amaranth being a close second.

And speaking of *amaranth*, this is a whole grain that has a cream of wheat like texture. Typically it's eaten as a breakfast cereal, but it can also be used like a polenta, mixed with gravies and sauces, and topped with sautéed vegetables.

Couscous, which I mentioned earlier, usually is used in place of rice alongside a major meal. It's also great with gravies and sauces.

Millet is also similarly used like cous cous and quinoa alongside of a major meal with gravies and sauces.

Now that we have gone over a variety of cooking preparation methods, meal preparation ideas, and different ways to prepare new and exciting grains and legumes, let's go back and review the anti-inflammatory diet. We're taking it back to basics. Generally, you want to get at least four to six servings of vegetables a day. That's the green leafy vegetables, broccoli, and red yellow and orange varieties of vegetables. These are the anti-inflammatory vegetables, and we'll go more into that soon enough. We want at least three fruit servings a day – berries and other high-antioxidant fruits are the key. Low-glycemic index foods, such as the good carbs which we discussed earlier, and our sugar alternatives – not Equal, not Splenda, not Sweet-N-Low, but stevia or agave nectar – those are the things that we want to concentrate on. In addition, get 25 to 35 grams of fiber per day. Fiber lowers the cholesterol; it also lowers the blood pressure.

So let's talk about the inflammatory foods a little bit more. We did talk about this before but we're reviewing now. Refined foods. Anything that's processed, white refined, is bound to cause inflammation, because the processing is so harsh and actually takes away the nutritional value of the food. Alcohol, fried foods, soft drinks, high fructose corn syrup, and many of the baked foods like cakes, are foods that need to be avoided and that cause inflammation to the body. In addition, your junk food snacks, like your Pringles or your potato chips, milk shakes, tobacco, MSG containing products, coffee drinks, and non-natural sugar substitutes as I just mentioned – Splenda, Equal, and Sweet-N-Low. How do you know some of these things? Read the labels. MSG also is called 'monosodium glutamate'. When you're picking out mixed spices or when you're picking up any type of canned or pre-prepared food, look at the label for any type of MSG or monosodium glutamate.

78

Also look at the label in your canned foods for high fructose corn syrup. If you see those ingredients, put it down and look for something that does not have those two ingredients in it.

Let's talk about the foods to limit – because we do things in moderation. You want to limit your dairy products, your red meats, your pork, poultry, and in general, your sugars. Sports drink, dried or preserved fruits – and this is because, when fruits are dried, they usually have added sugar. You want to limit your nuts (except for almonds, you can eat those freely). Limit your breads, pastas, whole egg yolks, stress (yeah, I know that's not a food, but I have to throw that in there!), your non-organic juices, and you want to limit soy.

I say to limit them, which means you don't have to completely eliminate them, but you want to eat them in moderation. What's moderation? The answer is occasionally, less than weekly or even once monthly if that. This is especially true of your red meat, your pork, and your poultry. Those meats do cause inflammation in the body and can clog up the digestive system. When the digestive system is clogged up, you don't, number one, get the proper elimination – and elimination is how we get rid of the toxins in our body – and in addition, you don't get the proper absorption of the nutrients needed to help the body function in its optimal way. So you really want to be aware. This is about conscious eating. This is about being aware of the type of foods you put in your body, so that you limit the inflammation that's going on and therefore halting and limiting the disease process.

Finally, we want to talk about the foods that you can enjoy, because there are plenty of foods that you can enjoy out there that are tasty and that are easy to prepare. All of your veggies you can enjoy – from your dark green leafies, to your red, your yellow, your orange variety – we talked about that earlier, but most definitely you want to enjoy all of the vegetables in great quantities.

When we talk about preparation of vegetables, it's best to eat them raw, but it's unrealistic to think that you're going to eat raw vegetables all the time. So the best preparation methods tend to be lightly steamed and stir fried, lightly stir fried. Otherwise, as long as you're getting the vegetables – and try to make them fresh vegetables. We talked a little bit about shopping and one thing that I may not have mentioned is that one of the best places to get your fresh vegetables is at the farmer's market, because the farmer's market does tend to have the fresh and locally grown as well as the organic vegetables and in addition, the farmer's market tends to be a little bit less expensive than your local grocer.

Fruits that you want to enjoy. As many fruits as you like, being careful of how sugary they are. You especially want to concentrate on your citrus fruits, your watermelons, your mango, your papaya, and your grapefruits. The reason papaya, pineapple, and those citrus fruits are great, because they're alkaline producing in the body and we talked earlier about how alkaline producing foods and alkaline foods decrease inflammation in the body, therefore promoting cellular health.

You want to also enjoy your seeds, like your sunflower or your pumpkin or hemp seeds. Not necessarily already prepared or roasted from the grocery store. You want to get them raw, and if you want to prepare them it's okay, but then you know how to prepare them yourself – sautéing them in a little olive oil, or a little ghee, rather than buying them prepared where you don't know how or what types of things have been added to the oils that have prepared or roasted your seeds.

We talked about whole grains, so you can enjoy your brown and wild rice. You can enjoy your quinoa, your millet, your barley, your amaranth. Flax seed is a great whole grain to enjoy because not only is it high in your omega acids, but it also is a great source of fiber.

Enjoy your herbal teas, especially green tea and red roobois, which is an African herbal tea. Your bomate is a great tea, but you want to be careful about how much you're eating because it has been shown in some studies to be linked to bladder cancer.

Fresh juices. I recommend going out and purchasing yourself

a juicer, and begin to get into juicing your own juices – juicing your own vegetables and fruits. A great juice that I like to prepare myself is a combination of spinach, apple, carrot, and ginger as well as celery. I prepare this juice and then I put just one small serving of stevia – one packet of stevia into the cup and it sweetens the juice so that it tastes like a regular juice out of the grocery store. There are definitely places where you can get your juices fresh. There are companies like Arden's Garden, Whole Foods which juice your fruits or vegetables for you right in front of you, and there are also brands out there that are 100% juice. But again, remember to read your labels and make sure that the juices do not have high fructose corn syrup and that they really are 100% juice and not necessarily from concentrate.

Enjoy your nuts, particularly almonds, hazelnuts, coconuts and Brazil nuts. Now I know I said to limit the nuts just earlier, but the ones you can enjoy are your almonds, hazelnuts, coconuts and Brazil nuts.

Can you enjoy Dark chocolate? – YES! The formal name being cacao, you can enjoy dark chocolate. It has many anti-inflammatory properties; it also helps the body produce something called nitrous oxide, which dilates the blood vessels. Image dilated blood vessels is very good for circulation and for the heart. It also helps to moderate or modulate the glycemic levels so you don't get those up and down sugar fluctuations in

82

the body. Also, dark chocolate curbs the sugar craving and can be bought in a variety of combinations, my favorite being dark chocolate and mint. Remember, if you're going to buy dark chocolate, buy at least 70%. Dark chocolate also helps to modulate certain neural transmitters in the brain like serotonin, so it can help with anxiety; it can also help with stress and depression. It's no substitute, if you have a moderate to severe depression, for going to your doctor, but just keep in mind that when you start to eat these foods that are anti-inflammatory in nature and that are healthy in nature, that have all these healing properties, you're going to decrease your chances of being stressed, depressed, and anxious overall.

I have a whole another series on balance that tackles stress and anxiety from the inside out, but this is just one approach.

Stevia, raw honey, agave nectar – those are your sugar substitutes or sugar sources that are safe to eat, that are anti-inflammatory in nature – or not inflammatory in nature, I should say. You can also enjoy your olive oil, your flax seed oil, your hemp oil, and your canola oil. Again, flax seed oil does have anti-inflammatory properties as does hemp and olive oil. And again, finally, your legumes – you can enjoy beans, lentils, and peas such as chickpeas.

Having gone over the anti-inflammatory foods, I also want to introduce some supplements that help to keep the inflammation down and that are heart-protective and just generally good for your health. Generally, a good vitamin and mineral supplementation is the key to proper function of the cells. A high potency multi-vitamin is a liquid vitamin by the Buried Treasure brand. It can be found in your local natural foods grocer or you can search it online. Coenzyme Q10 is another supplement that lowers the blood pressure. It is anti-inflammatory in nature and is shown to be protective of the heart.

Omega 3-6-9 supplement – typically the Omega 3-6-9 supplement contains fish oils, barrage seed oil, and flax seed oil. It can also contain hemp or evening primrose oil in the vegetarian preparations. The Omega 3-6-9 lowers cholesterol, is anti-inflammatory in nature, and also is great for skin conditions such as exema or scorisis. You can purchase the Omega 3-6-9 supplement in capsules in break them open or you can purchase them in a liquid supplement and apply it topically to your skin conditions such as exema or scorisis and it will improve that, because, again, they are natural anti-inflammatories.

Garlic capsules' transfer factor, which is a key component in colostrums, IP-6, also called inoxetol hexophosphate, green tea – those are all anti-inflammatory supplements that are great, especially for people who have conditions like fibromyalgia, lupus, or any other inflammatory-based condition. If you're healthy, just having a multi-vitamin, an omega supplement, and a super food supplement (which I'm about to go over) is enough. But for people who suffer from chronic fatigue, fibromyalgia, lupus, or any other autoimmune disorder, should definitely have things like transfer factor, inoxetol hexophosphate, and the green tea extracts on board.

So let's go back over your super food supplements. Super food supplements are like traditional vegetables but they have great properties of healing, such as wheat grass, barley grass, chlorella, alfalfa grass, and spirolina. These supplements have been known to create great healing properties in the body. They decrease inflammation, they increase the immune system, they detoxify the body, they balance the intestinal system, and many other things that they have been studied to do. There is a great product out there called Green Vibrance that contains all of these super food supplements and more.

Many of these super food supplements are great for lowering blood pressure, cholesterol, sugar, and decreasing the overall inflammation in the cells and in the body.

So now that we have gone over thoroughly different cooking methods, preparation methods, the anti-inflammatory diet, and even super food supplements, I want to give you a few quick recipes to start you out.

Breakfast

I'm going to start you out with a few basic breakfast ideas.

Let's start with a weekday breakfast. If you like oatmeal, then do an oatmeal (which is not instant) with a fruit of your choice. I like to either add blueberries, strawberries, or bananas to my oatmeal. You can even add a little almond to give it a crunchy flavor. Another quick and easy breakfast is to scramble an egg white and broil a piece of turkey bacon, and then add it to a toasted whole-grain piece of bread. Adding fruit into the yogurt of your choice with a high fibre, dry cereal is another quick and delicious breakfast treat. An example would be a plain, low-fat yogurt with half a cup of Total and a handful of blueberries. It's a quick, easy and healthy breakfast on the go.

Smoothies. All you need to do for a great smoothie is take the fruit of your choice, buy it in advance, and throw it in the freezer. So you may have a banana that you can peel, cut, and put in a freezer bag, strawberries, blueberries, already frozen. Take them, put them in your blender, add about a half a cup of water, one teaspoon of wheat germ, one teaspoon of honey, and maybe one eighth of a teaspoon of stevia, just to sweeten a little bit more, and blend it up – and you have a wonderful smoothie. You can also add a vegetable-based protein powder or super food supplement to get your vegetables in. Remember, I told you two vegetables each meal – so one great way to get your vegetables in is to throw it in your smoothie. You can throw a

86

handful of spinach in, or you can throw a super food powder like the Green Vibrance I told you about, into your fruit smoothie, and it won't taste any differently.

Pancake/Waffles

When you're indulging on the weekends for breakfast, consider a pancake or a waffle, whole grain prepared, with fresh fruit topping instead of syrup. You can also use a grade A, pure maple syrup, which has a lot more nutritional value than your Aunt Jemima's or your Log Cabin.

Another idea is whole grain French toast with a fruit topping, or homemade hash browns, baked instead of fried, with an omelet. How you make homemade hash browns is very easy. All you have to do is take a red potato or a creamer potato, and grate it. Add a little olive oil to the skillet and pan sear it and make a healthy hash brown.

Lunch/Dinner Ideas

Broccoli Casserole

- ✓ Here is a great recipe for a quick broccoli chicken casserole. Take one cup of dry brown rice to two cups of water.
- ✓ Begin boiling.
- ✓ Take two and a half cup of chicken breast (organic, with-

out the skin), chopped and cooked.

✓ Take a half a cup of onions, ten ounces of broccoli.

✓ Then take ten and three ounces of cream of mushroom soup (organic, buy the carton), one half cup of skim milk or almond milk if you're lactose intolerant, and a half a cup of fat free swiss cheese or even mozzarella, jarlesborg light, or the light cheese of your choice.)

✓ Take one teaspoon of basil and two tablespoons of tea salt, and a quarter teaspoon of black pepper.

You combine all of those elements, the cooked rice, the cooked chicken breasts, the chopped onions, the raw broccoli, the cream of mushroom soup, the milk, the cheese, and the spices, and you preheat the oven to 350. Put them all in a casserole dish and bake for approximately 20 minutes, covered. It's low in calories, low in fat, high in protein and low in sodium.

Another quick recipe is linguini and scallops, one of my favorites.

✓ Put the linguini on to boil and simultaneously go ahead and heat up your olive oil with a little garlic in it.

✓ Once the oil is hot and the garlic is browning, you may go ahead and add your scallops, while you're boiling your linguini.

- ✓ Within five to ten minutes, your scallops and your linguini should be done.
- ✓ Pour the linguini into a pan.
- ✓ Once the scallops are done, add a little bit of organic mushroom soup.
- ✓ Pour that sauce on top of the linguini and sprinkle a little bit of Parmesan Romano dry grated cheese over the top and mix well.

This is a great, quick Italian dish. Another version of this linguini with scallops is to use the fresh or frozen scallops with one teaspoon of margarine or ghee, one and a half cup of chicken broth, three tablespoons of lemon juice, three quarter cup of fresh parsley, two tablespoons of drained capers, one tablespoon of olive oil or cooking oil, three fourth cups of dry white wine or Vermouth, three-fourth cup of sliced green onion, one teaspoon of dill weed, and one teaspoon of pepper. Start the scallops, sautéing them in ghee, and while that's going on, stir the broth, white wine or cooking vermouth, and lemon juice into a skillet, bringing it to boil for about 10-12 minutes. Then reduce the heat and stir in the onions, parsley, caper, and dill weed. Once the scallops are done, add the sauce to the scallops and toss gently.

The next recipe is one of my favorites – it's Cajun jambalaya.
- ✓ You'll need boneless chicken, seafood or, if you are

89

vegetarian, a meat substitute like Seitan;

✓ one half large onion;

✓ a bell pepper;

✓ four cloves of garlic;

✓ five cups of water;

✓ three tablespoons of salt;

✓ one half teaspoon of cayenne pepper,

✓ three bay leaves,

✓ six ounces of tomato paste (organic),

✓ one pound of peeled shrimp, and

✓ two cups of brown rice.

In a separate pot you want to add the two cups of brown rice to the four cups of water and bring it to a boil. Meanwhile, you want to sauté your chicken or begin sautéing your shrimp, scallops or whatever seafood that you'd like until they're cooked and browned. You then add the water, the salt, the cayenne, the bay leaf, and the tomato paste, bringing it to a boil with the lid on. When the water is boiled, you add the shrimp last and brown rice. Stir it to a low fire and let it simmer, stirring every five minutes until the rice is fully cooked. This jambalaya can be done vegetarian as well and still taste just as good.

Finally, I want to give you a low-cal homemade chip recipe

as a healthy snack. What you'll need is one unpeeled baking potato and two tablespoons of fat free Italian dressing. Preheat your oven to 500 Fahrenheit. Lightly spray a cooking sheet with vegetable cooking spray or olive oil. Sliced the unpeeled baking potato into very thin slices. In a bowl, toss the potato slices with the dressing until evenly coated. Arrange potatoes in a single layer on the cookie sheet. Bake for about 20 minutes or until lightly browned on both sides, turning once after ten minutes. As a variation, you can sprinkle a little parmesan cheese on top for added taste.

So now that we've give you a couple of recipes to start you out, it's your turn to practice planning. Stop the CD and plan for a whole day's worth of meals for you or for the family. First, plan for a weekday – breakfast, lunch, snacks, and dinner. Then plan for the weekend. See how you do. Remember, healthy eating, healthy shopping and healthy cooking are a process. You have plenty of time to review this – you can listen to it over and over again to get the principles down and apply them to your own life.

7

Six Small Meals

Ideally, our bodies are made for grazing. Six small meals a day – that's breakfast, mid-morning snack, lunch, mid-afternoon snack, a light dinner, and then a light bedtime snack. This bonus section is a montage of different quick, fun, and easy recipes. Six each for breakfast, lunch, dinner, and then six snack recipes. Let's start with breakfast.

Six great breakfast ideas that we're going to go over include smoothies, oatmeals, amaranth hot cereal, quinoa hot cereal, egg breakfast sandwich and a breakfast burrito. Let's start with the first recipe for smoothies.

Smoothies are a wonderful, easy and quick way to get a

breakfast when you're running out the door. Many of us are very busy and a lot of people don't like to eat breakfast, but breakfast is one of the most important meals of the day. It gets the metabolism going. So if you're one of these people who doesn't like to eat breakfast or who is too busy to eat breakfast and wants to eat breakfast on the run, then smoothies is the thing for you. I've composed six different smoothie recipes that are easy and fun for you to just throw into the blender and go on your way.

Here's a helpful hint before we get started. A lot of these smoothies are fruit recipes. What I suggest is that you buy the fruit in advance, cut it up if need be, and freeze it so that all you need to do is take the fruit out of the freezer, throw it in the blender, add just a little water, and then blend it and you're on your way. It also gives the smoothie that nice, icy taste, rather than a creamy, milky taste.

I don't really have any names for these smoothies, so feel free to put a name or an identity to each of these smoothies.

Smoothie #1
- ✓ five strawberries,
- ✓ one peeled and cut kiwi,
- ✓ one half banana,
- ✓ one cup of peaches,
- ✓ one teaspoon of wheat germ,

✓ one tablespoon of honey, and

✓ one cup of cold water.

Again, take the frozen version of these fruits, throw them in the blender, and high-power blend it – and then you've got a 16 oz smoothie that you can take with you for breakfast and even drink a little along the way for a mid-morning snack.

Smoothie #2.

✓ five strawberries,

✓ a half a cup of mangoes,

✓ a half a cup of cherries,

✓ one cup of peaches,

✓ one teaspoon of wheat germ,

✓ one tablespoon of honey, and

✓ one cup of cold water.

Notice in this one I got a little topical – I love to add exotic fruits. So you can add any fruit of your own, I'm just giving you some options. If you like papaya, add that. If you like coconut, which will be in one of our other recipes, add that. And remember that you can add almonds if you like, or any other nut to kind of give it that nutty taste. I like to add the wheat germ because it gives it a little bit of protein and you can also add your own whey protein powder if you like, sometimes I do that, or a fiber supplement to give it a little bit more substance and a little bit more stick and stay.

Smoothie #3.

- ✓ Add a half a cup of blueberries,
- ✓ a half a cup of cherries,
- ✓ one mango,
- ✓ a half a banana,
- ✓ one cup of peaches,
- ✓ one teaspoon of wheat germ,
- ✓ one tablespoon of honey, and
- ✓ one cup of cold water.

I add the honey because it gives it a sweet, but that sort of honey, tangy flavor. And again, the wheat germ for that added protein and it gives it somewhat of a nutty flavor. One other thing you can add to your smoothies is flax seed or flax seed meal. This also gives it the omega 3 acids that you need and gives it somewhat of a nutty flavor. It also adds a little bit of protein as well. Here's another helpful hint: if you have as much of a sweet tooth as I do, you may want to add an additional 1/8 teaspoon of stevia, to sweeten it up just a little bit more.

Yet another hint: whenever you're making smoothies with

blueberries, you do not want to let it sit for any length of time, because, for some reason, blueberries congeal when they sit. So when you're making a smoothie out of blueberries, go ahead and drink it within the first hour or so.

Smoothie #4.
- ✓ A half a cup of blueberries,
- ✓ a half a cup of cherries,
- ✓ five strawberries,
- ✓ one half banana,
- ✓ one teaspoon of wheat germ,
- ✓ one tablespoon of honey, and
- ✓ one cup of cold water.

Again, you see how I'm keeping it simple. I like particular fruits that I add into my smoothies, and you'll come to know what fruits that you like in yours.

Smoothie#5
- ✓ Take one mango,
- ✓ one half cup of young, raw, coconut - (that's not the shredded kind, that's the raw young coconut that you can buy at any farmer's market),
- ✓ one half cup of pineapple,

✓ one half banana,

✓ one teaspoon of wheat germ,

✓ one teaspoon of flax seed,

✓ one tablespoon of honey and

✓ one cup of cold water.

Again, blend it up and if you need to add a little ice to make it a little bit icier, then you may do so.

Finally, Smoothie #6,

✓ is one mango,

✓ one kiwi,

✓ one cup of pineapple,

✓ one half banana, and

✓ one cup of spinach.

✓ one teaspoon of wheat germ,

✓ one tablespoon of honey,

✓ one teaspoon of flax seeds, and

✓ one cup of cold water.

Notice I added this time the spinach, and which spinach adds that vegetable into your breakfast, you can't really taste it in the smoothie itself. So experiment with adding some carrot or spinach into your smoothies. The carrot actually sweetens the smoothie just a little bit, and the spinach gives you that dark green look to it, but you can't really taste it and you get your dark green vegetable in the morning. Remember, in previous episodes, we said we need four to six vegetables a day. This is a great way to get one of those servings in right at the breakfast.

Again, keep in mind you can also add to your smoothies protein powder of any flavor (like a berry flavor or a vanilla flavor or even a chocolate flavor), you can add flax seed meal, almonds are great, you can even add almond butter or peanut butter to give it a little protein, a little stick and stay and a little bit of that nutty flavor, if you like. I even add a little flax seed oil in at times to make it smoother in texture. Now go and create your own smoothie with your favorite fruits.

Let's move on to the next thing, which are cereals, particularly hot cereals. As I'm recording this, we're in the month of October going into November so it's getting hot, and that's why I'm focusing more on the warm cereals. There are three different grains that I'm going to talk about in terms of making warm or hot cereals. That's oatmeal, amaranth, and quinoa. Now, oatmeal is a classic and I recommend buying the five-minute cook oatmeal rather than the instant oatmeal because the instant oatmeal typically has a lot of sugars and other preservatives added.

So let's start with oatmeal.

- ✓ take one and a half cup of water and
- ✓ combine w/three-quarters cup of oatmeal, rolled oats (we'll prepare it for a serving, if you want to double the serving you'll double the ingredients here)
- ✓ add a dash of salt,
- ✓ a teaspoon of cinnamon or allspice to the water.
- ✓ Now bring it all to a boil for about 15 min

Some people add their oatmeal to the water after it begins to boil, but I find that adding the oatmeal at the same time, before it begins to boil, actually gives the oatmeal a very smooth, rich flavor. In addition, in the water, I add about a teaspoon of flax seed oil to smooth things out. Once you boil the oatmeal for about fifteen minutes and it boils down into a porridge, I add a fruit of my choice. I love to add strawberries, blueberries, apples, or bananas while it's still warm so that it cooks into the oatmeal. Then afterwards I'll add golden raisins and/or almonds. This adds a little crunchy texture to it. Other things that you can add to your oatmeal are granola and flax seeds or wheat germ. Again, that adds somewhat of a nutty taste to it and adds a little bit of texture.

You will find that different varieties of grains that you can prepare in this manner alone are oat grouts or steal cut oats instead of the rolled oats. And then you can use amaranth grain and quinoa. Amaranth is like a cream of wheat, so if you're a fan of a more smooth texture hot cereal, or if you just want a variety, you can use the same recipe that I just mentioned but prepare it with amaranth grain instead of oatmeal, or even cream of wheat if you like that. Amaranth grain has more protein and more stick and stay than your typical cream of wheat, but cream of wheat is just as well.

Again, quinoa, which is just thicker than amaranth but a little bit finer than oatmeal and has a distinct texture about it, can be prepared the same way as I mentioned the oatmeal, with a dash of salt and cinnamon or allspice as well as the one teaspoon of flax seed oil added to the water and boiled. The same proportions apply to amaranth and quinoa as oatmeal – two parts water to one part grain. Both quinoa, amaranth and oatmeal are all very easy and quick to prepare.

Alright, let's move on to a scrambled egg sandwich. This is so easy to prepare in the morning and, again, it gives you your protein and gives you your stick and stay so that you don't get famished before lunch. The scrambled egg sandwich can be done in a variety of ways but the simplest way to do it is to just take:

✓ two whole eggs or two whole egg whites,

✓ scramble them, add your favorite spice – maybe sea salt with a little bit of dill or chives or whatever it is that you like to put in your egg, lemon pepper is also a great added spice to the scrambled egg –

✓ and then, once scrambled in the fashion that you like it,

✓ Add it to a whole-wheat piece of toast with a slice of turkey bacon and maybe sprinkle some cheese of your choice on top.

I like to do the bread, the turkey bacon, scramble the cheese into the eggs, and put that on the piece of toast. You can also put it on a whole wheat bagel or a croissant. This is three different varieties of the same meal.

The next breakfast item that includes eggs is the breakfast burrito scramble. This is a little bit more indulgent, but it still doesn't take more than ten minutes to prepare.

✓ Scramble your eggs with

✓ onions,

✓ tomato,

✓ garlic,

✓ spinach,

✓ and optionally ground chicken, ground turkey, or even

turkey bacon.

Once you've scrambled all that together, just wrap it in a low-carb or whole-wheat tortilla. This is a very high protein, filling, and very portable breakfast for those days when you're on the go.

So we've covered a variety of breakfast foods from smoothie to hot cereal to egg varieties and now we're going to move on to lunches. The first and most simple thing that we're going to talk about is a different sandwich.

The first sandwich that we're going to talk about is just as simple as a PB&J, except we're going to use almond butter. Let's do an almond butter spread onto a piece of whole wheat toast, drizzle a little honey, and put the second piece of bread on. It's that simple. You can also use jam and you can put bananas on top if you like bananas – almond butter and banana sandwich. Some people may frown on this, but it's a simple, easy, on–the-go, high protein sandwich and you can eat it with a fruit cup.

The second sandwich is more of a wrap. This is a classic deli wrap, which can be done with meat or without meat.

✓ Take your whole wheat or low-carb tortilla and
✓ Add small broccoli heads,

- ✓ sprouts,
- ✓ shredded carrots,
- ✓ the meat (like a shredded chicken or even a deli turkey) of your choice, (if you're a vegetarian you can just do the veggies, or you can add a tofu)
- ✓ chopped tomatoes, and then
- ✓ the salad dressing of your choice (I recommend either an Italian, French, or a thousand-islands style dressing.)

Wrap it up and you're good to go for a great, easy, deli wrap.

The next type of sandwich is more of a wrap as well, is a lettuce wrap. Lettuce wraps are very easy and very healthy. I hardly even put iceberg lettuce in recipes, but this is the case where iceberg lettuce is actually very useful.

- ✓ Take an iceberg lettuce head, and take one iceberg leaf off, prepared shredded chicken.
- ✓ chopped tomatoes, and
- ✓ chopped mushrooms

To prepare the chicken: Take a chicken breast, cook it (either broil or pan sear), then you'll tear it apart with two forks after it's cooked. Sprinkle it with a little bit of Bragg's Liquid Aminos or, if you don't have that, you can use soy sauce, let it marinate. Put the chopped tomatoes, chopped mushrooms, and chicken in the lettuce leave and wrap it up and you have yourself a wonderful lettuce wrap.

Keep in mind, you're not limited to the vegetables that I add into the lettuce wrap. Feel free to create your own lettuce wrap using the base that I talked here, and then adding your own variety of vegetables.

Let's move on to salads. I've got six salad recipes that are easy to make and fun to eat. Keep in mind that any of these recipes can be used with or without meat. Also, keep in mind that if you take your salad, place it in a Tupperware, and then place just the right amount of salad dressing in (a serving is usually two tablespoons), you can shake it up and distribute all of the dressing so that you're not over utilizing the dressing and the salad remains healthy. Another tip is, with salad dressings, to have it on the side – then you can take each salad bite and dip it, getting the taste of the salad dressing, but again not overdoing it and destroying the nutritional value of the salad itself.

Salad option #1 (which is my favorite, low fat Caesar).

✓ Take romaine,

- ✓ two cups of romaine,
- ✓ one chopped roma tomato or you can use a half a cup of grape tomatoes,
- ✓ five or six olives,
- ✓ a teaspoon of capers, and
- ✓ then grated parmesan

Add a light Caesar or a light Parmesan dressing on top, and shake into the salad. Again, you can add chicken or one of my favorites is to blacken some salmon.

To blacken the salmon: take a little bit of olive oil onto a skillet, turn the burner to medium fire, sprinkle some Cajun seasoning over both sides of the salmon filet, and then just blacken it. Just put it on the pan hot and wait until the pink salmon starts to turn a little bit lighter. Flip it and again, just cook it a matter of five minutes and you have yourself a blackened Caesar salad. You can blacken chicken in the same way, you just have to cook the chicken a little bit longer.

Salad #2 - spring salad.

- ✓ This I love to do in March, April – thus a 'spring salad' – because it contains a lot of the fruits that I love.

- ✓ take two cups of romaine,
- ✓ about a half a cup to a cup of grape tomatoes,
- ✓ a half a cup of strawberries,
- ✓ a quarter cup of blueberries,
- ✓ a quarter cup of kiwis,
- ✓ one half apple, chopped,
- ✓ about a quarter cups of almond slivers, and
- ✓ then sprinkle about a quarter cup of feta or blue cheese crumbles and top and
- ✓ a raspberry vinaigrette dressing.

Again, a very good protein source to add is either a baked chicken or a baked tofu if you're vegetarian.

Salad Option # 3 traditional chef's salad.

- ✓ Use either romaine, green leaf lettuce, or baby spin-ach.
- ✓ Take two cups of either of these types of lettuce,
- ✓ add in about one half cup, chopped roma or yellow tomato,
- ✓ one chopped, broiled egg,
- ✓ five to six olives,
- ✓ one half cup of chopped mushrooms (either baby bella

or traditional button mushrooms)

✓ one to two slices of your favorite deli meat, (chicken or turkey.)

Roll the piece of turkey and then you slice it and lay it on top of your salad. Then top your salad with a creamy Italian light, or you can top it with a creamy thousand island or a French. These are three great low calorie dressings that can go on any chef's salad.

Salad option # 4 Asian spinach salad.

✓ take five cups of fresh spinach,

✓ one cup of bean sprouts,

✓ two clementines (peeled and segmented),

✓ one third cup of sliced fresh mushrooms,

✓ a third cup of vegetable oil,

✓ two tablespoons of soy sauce, and

✓ a pinch of garlic powder.

To make the salad dressing: in a small bowl you whisk to-gether the oil, the soy sauce, and the garlic powder. Then combine the spinach, the bean sprouts, the clementines, and the fresh mushrooms, and pour the dressing mixture over the salad.

107

Shake up to distribute evenly. I love this recipe actually, it's very light, but very good. And again, you can add chicken or tofu to give yourself a protein source and to give this salad a little stick and stay.

Salad #6: Another type of salad that you can use is a pasta salad. This salad is a feta and spinach pasta salad.

- ✓ Take one pound of spiral or small shelled pasta,
- ✓ a half pound of crumbled feta,
- ✓ two packages of frozen spinach or two cups of fresh spinach,
- ✓ one can of black olives, drained, or a bottle of green olives,
- ✓ two medium tomatoes, diced,
- ✓ one tablespoon of finely chopped mint,
- ✓ one half cup of olive oil,
- ✓ two tablespoons of red wine vinegar,
- ✓ three tablespoons of fresh lemon juice,
- ✓ one clove of crushed garlic,
- ✓ one teaspoon of finely chopped oregano.

Cook the pasta according to package directions, steam spinach in just the water that clings to it for a few minutes in a tightly covered saucepan. Remove from the heat after the spin-ach wilts, then toss the spinach into the pasta, top with the tomatoes and olives, and then combine the rest of the ingredients (the red wine vinegar, the lemon juice, the crushed garlic and the finely chopped oregano) and pour over the salad. You top the salad, then, with the crumbled feta cheese and serve. This recipe that I just named serves four people, so if you like to just make it for yourself, then you just quarter the recipe. But I suggest go-ing ahead and making the recipe for four and then you can have a couple of days' worth.

Finally, Salad #6 Bean salad. This recipe has a mediterraneal feel to it.

- ✓ Start with two organic cans of black beans, poured into a bowl.
- ✓ add one cup of fresh chopped cilantro,
- ✓ add the juice of one lemon and one lime,
- ✓ one half chopped yellow onion,
- ✓ two chopped cloves of garlic, and
- ✓ one chopped roma tomato.

Into the two cans of black beans, add the onion, the tomato, the garlic, and the cilantro, and then we'll juice the lemon and the lime, add a quarter cup of olive oil, whisk well and then pour that over the black beans. Toss the liquid into the black beans so that it's evenly distributed, and then you can let it marinate in the refrigerator for about 15 to 20 minutes and it's ready to serve. If you like Mediterranean flavor, this is a wonderful salad.

To go with these sandwiches and salads that we talked about, you might want a soup variety. So let's talk about a couple of soup recipes. This first recipe is one of my favorites to make because it's so simple and easy.

Cream of broccoli soup.

You'll need:

- ✓ eight cups of vegetable broth,
- ✓ one tub of tofutti sour cream or low-fat traditional sour cream,
- ✓ three-fourth cup chopped onion,
- ✓ three-fourth cup chopped celery,
- ✓ one tablespoon of sea salt,
- ✓ a pinch of ground white pepper,
- ✓ two cups of almond milk or low fat skimmed milk (organic),
- ✓ one third cup of corn starch,
- ✓ one fourth cup of water,
- ✓ three cups of fresh broccoli florets, and
- ✓ one and a half cups of shredded Colby cheese.

In a saucepan, combine the broth, the onion, the celery, the salt, and the pepper, bring to a boil. Reduce the heat, cover and simmer for five to ten minutes. Then, in a small bowl, mix corn starch and the water until the corn starch is completely dissolved. Then gradually add the mixture to the soup, stirring constantly. Add the broccoli fluorites. Allow that to boil for five to ten minutes longer. Then add the milk, followed by sprinkling over of the cheddar cheese, gradually, until it's all melted into the soup. Once you've completed this step, next you'll add in the tofurgy sour cream or your low fat sour cream, and you'll stir to make it creamy. At this point you need to turn the eye down to low, cover, and simmer for about fifteen minutes. This soup recipe is delicious, but it's often even better the next day.

Let's go on to another soup recipe that's an old family favorite: Leek Cream of Potato Soup.
- ✓ start with three leeks,
- ✓ four red potatoes, quartered,
- ✓ a quarter cup of ghee,
- ✓ a half cup of low fat organic milk or unsweetened original almond milk,
- ✓ almond milk,
- ✓ a half cup of tofutti sour cream or low fat traditional sour

cream,

- ✓ one quart of water or vegetable stock,
- ✓ one quarter teaspoon of chopped cilantro,
- ✓ two tablespoons of chopped celery and
- ✓ 1/4 cup shallots,
- ✓ one-eighth teaspoon of celery seed, and
- ✓ parsley to garnish.

You can either peel the red potatoes, or you can leave the skin on. I prefer to leave the skin on the red potato, because therein lies some of the nutrients and it gives it actually more of a texture. Prepare the leeks by removing the green portion, preserving for other use if desired. Cut down the center, lengthwise, and wash thoroughly. Chop the white portions finely and sauté lightly with the chopped salad and half of the ghee for five to seven minutes. Then add one quart of water or vegetable stock, add one half teaspoon of sea salt, celery, the quartered potatoes, and simmer for 20 minutes. Remove the potatoes and leeks to a small bowl. Using a potato masher, mash to a puree and return the puree to the cooking water. Stir in the milk or almond milk, the sour cream or tofurgy sour cream, and the remaining ghee, reheating one minute if needed. Season to taste with the salt and the pepper, and garnish with the cilantro and parsley. This is an absolute favorite in the wintertime, and because it serves at least six you can eat it for more than one day for lunch – just put it in a Tupperware. You might even combine it with a salad or a sandwich and you've got a quick brown-bag lunch that you can warm up right at your desk.

Other great and easy soup recipes are cream of tomato soup and cream of mushroom soup. These are things that you can buy in the store already prepared and at the end of this segment, I'll give you a couple of websites where you might be able to find homemade cream of mushroom or cream of tomato recipes. But for now, we're going to move on to healthy dinners.

If you're anything like me, when you come home from a long day's work you're tired, and the last thing you want to do is slave over some stove for dinner. To tell you the truth, some days I come home and have a bowl of cereal and call it a day. But on a normal day, when I'm trying to live my healthy lifestyle, trying to live my creed, I have come up with some great meals that are easy to prepare in less than 30 minutes. This is also something you can do for the family, because it's easy for someone who's single to come home and eat a bowl of cereal or a piece of cheese toast, but when you're not alone it's clear that you have more than yourself to think about.

Dinner recipe #1

Let's get started with our first meal, which is a Veggie or Meat Stir Fry. This meal is easy because it only takes three to four steps – three steps if you're cooking it vegetarian style, four steps if you're cooking it with meat. If you're cooking your stir-fry with meat, you want to start by putting the rice on to boil.

Starting the Rice & Chicken Preparations:

- ✓ Take two parts water to one part rice – (for example, if you put three cups of water on, then you need to put one and a half cup of brown rice.) Go ahead and put the water and the rice in and bring to a boil. Once it's boiling, turn the heat down to medium.
- ✓ The next thing you'll do if you're cooking with chicken is go ahead and put it on to pan sear. Take one tablespoon of olive oil and put it over a medium heat skillet. Then you'll take your chicken, unseasoned, and put it on medium heat to pan sear.
- ✓

Preparing Seafood:
- ✓ Add two tablespoons of olive oil to your wok over medium heat.
- ✓ Next add your chopped garlic and
- ✓ chopped onion and sauté until lightly brown.

114

✓ add your scallops or shrimp, or both if you like, to the pot and

✓ sauté until they're lightly brown.

You'll know when the seafood is done as the scallops do have a light golden color and the shrimp will turn from a clear look to more of a whitish look and will be lightly browned.

While you're doing this, you can go ahead and begin to prepare your veggies.

✓ Take out one half pound of snap peas,

✓ two cups of bean sprouts,

✓ two cloves of garlic,

✓ a quarter of an onion to chop,

✓ one half cup watercress,

✓ two cups broccoli, and

✓ one cup sliced carrots.

Keeping a watch on your chicken, turning when necessary, you'll want to go ahead and start by snapping your peas and breaking them in half, chopping your garlic finely, chopping your quarter onion (mediumly fine), slicing your carrots or alternatively, when you purchase them, they can be already sliced, and taking your broccoli off the stalks.

Alternatively, you can buy frozen vegetable stir-fry with the vegetables already prepared. Another alternative, to cut down on steps, is instead of cooking your chicken you can purchase already cooked chicken breast and already cooked shrimp or scallops if you choose to make your stir-fry with seafood. At this point, if you're preparing your meat from scratch, your chicken should be already done. You'll take it off of the burner and set it to the side. At this point add the rest of your vegetables – your snap peas, your bean sprouts, your watercress, your broccoli, and your sliced carrots.

Lightly sauté them for five to ten minutes. Then add a quarter to half a cup of Bragg's Liquid Amino Acids (or soy sauce if you don't have the Bragg's) to the mixture to give it that more Asian taste. You can also add one quarter of a cup of teriyaki sauce if you want your vegetables to have a little bit sweeter of a flavor. Sauté just a little bit longer, turn the heat to low, and you're ready to serve. By this time your brown rice should be well cooked, but keep in mind that you will need to watch over it as you're preparing this recipe and stir it every and now and again. If you're cooking with the chicken, you've already stir fried your vegetables without the seafood, go ahead and chop up the meat and add it to the seafood after you've sautéed the vegetables for the five to ten minutes. Then add the Bragg's

116

Liquid Amino Acids and/or the teriyaki sauce and your meal will be ready to serve within five minutes.

Now let's move on to another quick and easy meal that takes less than 20 minutes to prepare.

Steamed Asparagus w/Mushroom Quinoa
- ✓ You'll need:
- ✓ one pound of steamed asparagus,
- ✓ one cup of quinoa grain,
- ✓ one cup of organic mushroom soup, and
- ✓ one to two sweet potatoes or, alternatively, you can use sweet yams.

Start by putting your quinoa on to boil. Take two parts water to one part quinoa – again, that would be three cups of water to one and a half cup quinoa or make the quantity to the specification of your needs. Go ahead and put the quinoa in the water before it begins to boil. Add one teaspoon of ghee or margarine if you don't have ghee, and when it comes to a boil turn the heat down to a medium. If you're on a boiler that's from 0 to 9, that would be turning it down to about a 5 or a 6. Keep an eye on this as you prepare the other items. Next thing you'll do is take your two yams, go ahead and put them in a pot and fill the pot with water just enough to cover the sweet potatoes or the yams. Bring it to a high boil and, once it's boiling, turn it down to a medium high heat. If you're boiler goes from 0 to 9, that would be about a 7 or 8. Let the potatoes boil for about 15 minutes. The quinoa will be finished in about 15 minutes. At about 15 minutes, when the quinoa is just getting done, you'll go ahead and start your steamed asparagus. You usually start the asparagus last because they take the least amount of time to cook and you don't want to overcook your vegetables. So what you will need for this is a large pot with a steam basket. You put the water into the bottom of the large pot and put your steam basket on top, placing the asparagus inside the basket. You can sprinkle a little salt on top of the asparagus prior to and maybe even put a little teaspoon of ghee on top for taste. Place the top on and turn the burner on high to bring the water to a boil. Once the water is at a boil, you can turn the boiler down to low immediately. The water will continue to boil and the steam will continue to cook the asparagus and even when the water stops boiling, the steam will continue to rise, further cooking the asparagus. My suggestion is, once you have turned the boiler off, go ahead and take the pot off of the hot boiler and allow the steam to naturally continue to cook the asparagus so the asparagus don't overcook. By this time, your quinoa should be ready. All you need to do is add a pinch of dill weed and your cup of mushroom sauce and you're ready to go. Your sweet potato, by this point, should be well boiled. Take the sweet potato off the boiler, run it under cold water, and peel the sweet potato (being very careful not to scald yourself!). Once the sweet potato is peeled, add one teaspoon of honey and one quarter cup of almond milk or a low-fat milk, and mash well. This is a complete meal in itself, but if you'd like to add meat to this meal, you can blacken a chicken breast or a salmon filet. All you would need to do is take that salmon filet, add a little lemon pepper, same thing with the chicken – take the chicken breast, add a little lemon pepper, add one tablespoon of olive oil to a medium-hot skillet, and pan sear. In this meal you'll get your complex carbohydrate, your protein source, your grain, and your vegetable. Please note that you would get your protein source whether or not you add the meat to the meal, because the quinoa is a very good source of protein.

Our next meal is an easy classic: Red Beans & Rice

Since typically red beans and brown rice take a little longer to cook, we're going to use a pressure cooker. This is a great investment because it allows a lot more variety than what would normally take longer to cook. If you know you're going to make your red beans and brown rice, you want to soak your beans that day before you go to work. So just take the beans, put them in a Tupperware filled with water (just enough to cover the beans), and put them in the refrigerator. When you come home they would have been sufficiently soaked.

The first stage in the preparation of the beans and rice is putting the beans in the pressure cooker to boil. You'll want to read the directions of your pressure cooker, but most pressure cookers have a mechanism that tells you when the pressure is elevated. Secondly, you'll want to read your pressure cooker's manual to know how long to leave the beans in, but for most you'll cook the beans for 30 minutes.

- ✓ Place three cups of water,
- ✓ a dash of salt, and
- ✓ Your previously soaked one-cup of dry beans into the mixture.

Seal the lid and turn on high. When the pressure indicator begins gently rocking, you will turn the boiler down to medium. Again, if you have a broiler that goes from 0 to 9, you'll put it down to about 5 to 6. The pressure indicator will continue to gently rock and as long as that's happening you have enough pressure to quickly cook your beans. '

Your next step is to put on your brown rice.

Add two parts water to one part rice. In this case, you'll want to add two cups of water and once cup of rice.

Bring it to a fast boil and, once the water is boiling, turn it down again to medium heat.

On your third boiler, we're going to make a sautéed okra and tomatoes combination.

- ✓ You'll take two garlic cloves, chop them finely;
- ✓ take a quarter of an onion, chopped finely, and
- ✓ a half a pound of okra and you'll chop that coarsely
- ✓ a roma tomato, cut in large chunks.

In your skillet, go ahead and put one teaspoon of ghee and allow it to melt into the pan. Add your chopped garlic and onion, sauté for two minutes. Then add your okra and sauté for another three to four minutes. Finally, add your cut tomatoes and stir until the mixture comes to a boil. You can add salt and pepper to taste. By this point your beans should be done, if about 20 to 30 minutes has passed. Take the pressure cooker off the burner. Place it in the sink and run cool water over the lid until the pressure indicator indicates that the pressure is lifted. Please read the instructions on your pressure cooker's manual as to different ways to release the pressure without burning yourself with the steam. You must take great care, because injury can occur if not careful.

Once the pressure is released from the pressure cooker, you

may open it. You'll add the okra and tomato mixture and the cooked brown rice and stir. Go ahead and add a seasoned salt to taste. For additional added flavor, you can add a cup of Ragu or Prego spaghetti sauce. This meal is high in protein, high in fiber, and has your vegetables alongside of it. It's an actual easy one, as well, to pack up and take to lunch the next day.

Moving on to the next meal, blackened salmon with a spicy brown rice and sautéed spinach. Take your blackened salmon and go ahead and season it with a Cajun seasoning on both sides and set it to the side. Next, place three cups of water to one and a half cup of rice or prepare to your specifications using two cups water to one cup rice. You'll go ahead and put salt and the same Cajun seasoning in the water to boil. As the rice comes to a boil, turn the burner down to medium heat. Next, go ahead and put two tablespoons of olive oil in your skillet and bring to a medium heat. Place your seasoned salmon on the medium heat skillet and allow it to pan sear for two to three minutes before turning. Allow it to pan sear for two to three minutes longer. At this point it should be done. You can remove it from the heat or turn the heat down to low and cover. On a third burner, you can begin to prepare your spinach. Take two cups of raw spinach, set it to the side. One clove of garlic and one roma tomato. Heat up two tablespoons of olive oil over medium heat and add your chopped garlic. Lightly sauté for two to three minutes or until golden brown and then add your spinach. Your spinach will begin to be coated with the oil. Continue to sauté, stirring lightly over the heat, until the spinach begins to wilt. Once the spinach is wilted, add your chopped tomato. Sauté for only two to three more minutes, turn the burner down to low, and cover, letting it simmer. By this time your rice should be done; salt it to taste. Serve the salmon over the rice and put the sautéed spinach on the side. Here you have your protein, your grain, and a tasty vegetable.

Let's move on to our next dinner, Lemon Pepper Chicken, broiled; Mashed Cauliflower; and Glazed Baby Carrots.

In this recipe your mashed cauliflower serves more like your mashed potato, but without the high carb content.

Lemon Pepper Chicken: To start, take your chicken breast, place it on a piece of foil that can be wrapped around it, drizzle one teaspoon of olive oil over the chicken breast. Add your lemon pepper and massage into the chicken. Add one garlic clove, chopped finely.

Wrap & Place on a cookie sheet and place into the oven. You'll turn your oven, preheated, to 300 degrees on broil, not bake. Set your timer for about 20 minutes.

Cauliflower Mashed potatoes: We're next going to prepare the cauliflower in a steamed fashion. As earlier mentioned, take your steamer, place the water in the bottom, your basket on top, placing the cauliflower in the steam basket and cover. Turn the boiler on high and bring the water to a boil. Allow your cauliflower to steam for 10 minutes. As your cauliflower is steaming, let's go on to the baby carrots.

Baby Carrots: Take one bag of raw baby carrots and place them in a saucepan. Fill the sauce pan with just enough water to cover the baby carrots. Turn the boiler on to medium heat and bring to a low boil. Once the water is boiling, immediately turn the boiler down to a low heat. We don't want to over boil the baby carrots. At this point, you're going to add one tablespoon of raw sugar into the water, cover, and let simmer for the next few minutes.

While your baby carrots are simmering we'll turn our attention back to the cauliflower, which should be fully steamed. Take the softened cauliflower out of the steam basket and place it in a plastic or Pyrex bowl. Add one tablespoon of margarine or ghee and begin to mash. You can also add just a slight bit of almond milk or you can add a low fat organic milk, an eighth of a cup at most, and mash until creamy. If you have a hand blender, this is a great tool to create a whipped feel to your mashed cauliflower. Once your cauliflower is mashed to a creamy substance, go ahead and salt and pepper to taste.

Now we have completed the mashed cauliflower and the glazed baby carrots, we want to check on our lemon pepper chicken. Stick a fork in the middle to make sure that it's fully cooked and if it is, take it out of the oven and serve.

Our final dinner is a new recipe that I've learned from a good friend of mine, Southwestern Chili.

For this you'll need:

- ✓ organic canned white corn,
- ✓ a half a pound of okra which you'll chop coarsely,
- ✓ four roma tomatoes which you'll cut into large chunks,
- ✓ two cups of red kidney beans,
- ✓ a pound of ground turkey or two cups of textured vegetable protein,

depending on whether you're preparing this chili with meat or vegetarian style. If you're preparing this vegetarian style, you'll need to soak the TVP, or textured vegetable protein.

TVP Preparation Method: Take the two cups of textured

vegetable protein, place it in enough water to cover at least an inch over the textured vegetable protein, add some chipotle seasoning to the water, cover and place in the refrigerator for an hour to two hours prior to preparing your meal.

For the preparation of the beans, you can either buy the organic canned, already cooked kidney beans or, if you're using dry kidney beans, we will soak them in the same method that we soaked the black beans when we made the red beans and rice. If we're preparing this chili with ground turkey,

- ✓ Take one tablespoon or two tablespoons of olive oil and place in a skillet over medium heat.
- ✓ Add a quarter chopped onions and
- ✓ one chopped clove of garlic.

Then add your ground turkey with a little chipotle seasoning sprinkled on top and begin to brown.

While your turkey is browning, go ahead and put three cups of water and your previously soaked kidney beans into the water with a little chipotle seasoning and a little bit of salt – just a teaspoon of salt in the water. Place the top onto the pressure cooker and put on to high heat until the pressure indicator begins to rock slightly. Again, when this happens, turn the heat down to medium heat and the pressure cooker will continue to rock gently. You will cook your kidney beans for about 30 minutes. Again, remember to read the manual for your pressure cooker to get the exact time needed to cook a soaked red kidney bean. While the beans are cooking, turn your attention back to the ground turkey and continue to brown.

If you're using TVP, at this point you will drain the water from the soaked TVP, place two tablespoons of olive oil to a skillet and begin to brown the TVP. Browning TVP is much like sautéing. You keep the skillet on medium heat, but you need to stir more constantly so that the textured vegetable protein does not burn. You'll know the textured vegetable protein is ready when it begins to slightly brown. In this case, it doesn't need to be dry, it just needs to be browned slightly. Once your TVP is done, turn on low heat, set to the side, and simmer. Also at this point if you're using ground turkey, it should be set to the side simmering as well. Once 30 minutes pass on the pressure cooker your kidney beans should be done cooking. Take the pressure cooker off the boiler, put it in the sink, run cool water over the top of the pressure cooker to release and equalize the pressure – again, read the manual for different methods of your pressure cooker releasing the pressure. Carefully open the lid of

the pressure cooker and then place the saucepan portion of the
pressure cooker back on the stovetop over low heat and add the
rest of the ingredients. You'll add your canned white organic
corn, your chopped okra, your tomatoes, and your ground turkey
or TVP. Stir in and add just a little bit more water, about one to
two cups, so that it gives a little bit of a soupy feel to it. Salt and
pepper to taste, and you have yourself a wonderful southwestern
chili. You might want to let simmer for another fifteen minutes,
just to let the seasonings seep into all of the vegetables and the
beans themselves. This is also a great meal to take the next day
for lunch.

Now that we've gotten six great dinner recipes in, I want to
turn our attention to snacks. I won't so much give you recipes
for snacks, but great snack ideas. I've done this in a previous
lecture – if you were part of the healthy cooking lecture then you
know some of the great snacks that we've already talked about.
But here are some that I haven't mentioned.

Snack number one: take five to six whole strawberries. Place
them in a ziplock bag, and take one teaspoon of raw sugar.
Place it as well in the ziplock bag, and shake. You can take this
to work with you and have it as a yummy, sweet snack. One of
the things I like about this snack is that it actually curbs the
sugar craving for those of you who have a sweet tooth, like I do.

Another unsuspecting snack is dark chocolate. Purchase a nice brand name of dark chocolate such as Ghirardelli, Lindt, or Velour, and what you would do is take two squares of that dark chocolate only and have it as a snack. The chocolate should be 70% dark or greater. You can buy a variety of combination dark chocolate such as chocolate mint, chocolate with almonds, chocolate with infused fruits such as pear or berries. It gives you a lot more variety to the snack. At any rate, the dark chocolate helps to curb the sweet craving and it also curbs the carb craving.

The next snack is apples and almond butter. This is a variation on a daycare classic, apples and peanut butter. It's easy – just chop your apple and spread a little almond butter on top and you have a healthy and tasty snack. A variation on the almond butter snack is a rice cake and almond butter. Rice cakes come in a variety of flavors. They come large and they come in little rice cake bites. Either way, you can spread almond butter on top of whatever flavor rice cake as you like and to add a little bit more of a sweet taste, you can add a half a teaspoon of honey to the top of the almond butter and swirl and you get a little sweet treat. The almond butter has protein and the rice cake is low calorie.

Another easy, fun snack recipe is trail mix – but not just your ordinary trail mix, a spicy trail mix! This is a recipe that I actually got from my father. You can take brazil nuts, walnuts, almonds, dried raisins, goji berries, dried cranberries, or dried cherries, or all of the above, place them into a large freezer bag, add a quarter teaspoon of sea salt, a half teaspoon of cumin powder, a quarter teaspoon of curry (yellow), a quarter teaspoon of turmeric, and shake. The seasonings will coat the contents and you'll have yourself a spicy trail mix. Alternatively you can use Jamaican dry spices or chipotle spices and the aforementioned nut mix to create your variety of spicy trail mix.

One final snack idea is to take a cup of plain yogurt, chop your favorite fruit up, and add it to the plain yogurt. And you can also add your favorite flavor granola, and you have a quick, tasty and healthy treat.

So we've given you six recipes each for breakfast, lunch, dinner and snacks. Keep in mind that these recipes are just templates from which you can employ your imagination to expand upon and even create your own recipes. To conclude this book (and in keeping with the "six" theme), I want to leave you with six recipe websites to explore to help you find your inner intuitive cook. Here they are.

The first website is www.glutnfreeda.com. For anyone who may have a restriction for gluten or wheat, this is a great website to explore. The second website is www.cooks.com. The third recipe website is www.allrecipes.com. The third recipe website is www.internationalrecipesonline.com. The next recipe website is www.recipe-source.com, and the final is www.stgabriel.net.

Many of these recipe websites have vegetarian, meat-based, and international recipes for any taste that you desire. I hope that you find these recipes useful. Please feel free to use to reference this book as many times as you need to integrate all of the information aforementioned in this book.

About the Author

Maiysha "Dr. Life" Clairborne MD the founder of Mind Body Spirit Wellness Inc. A board certified Family Physician and with nearly a decade of experience, Dr. Clairborne detoured from western medicine due to her dissatisfaction with the limitations of her traditional degree. Having landed herself in the world of integrative medicine, today she focuses her practice in the areas of natural disease management, emotional wellness, sexual health, and stress reduction. Her office services include acupuncture, holistic life coaching, clinical nutrition management, and mind body techniques , however, Dr. Clairborne offers a variety of Mind Body Wellness programs for people nationwide.

An internationally traveled speaker, facilitator, and wellness coach, Dr. Clairborne's passion shows in both her practice and in the community. Every day, she changes hundreds of people's perspective on exercise and healthy eating. She motivates and encourages dozens to set boundaries for themselves in order to balance their life and reduce their stress. She helps others to remember their own worth. She simplifies lifestyle change so that proper eating and getting or staying active feels manageable enough for them to take that first step. She shares in her books, lectures, and retreats her most successful strategies to in order to improve diseases that other doctors may not have been able to manage through the basic principles of functional nutrition and proper supplementation. All of this she does while maintaining a lifestyle congruent with her teachings. She has been featured on shows such as the CW's Focus Atlanta, Sacramento & Company, NBC40 Health Update, and Rx for Life. Her expert articles appear in the DermaScope Magazine and Lovegevity ongoing relationship column. Dr. Maiysha Clairborne is also the host of the streaming radio show The Wellness Dialogues.

Eat Your Disease Away References:

Food as Medicine: *How to Use Diet, Vitamins, Juices, and Herbs for a Healthier, Happier, and Longer Life*, Dharma Singh, M.D. Khalsa, Atria (January 6, 2004)

Healing with Whole Foods: Asian Traditions and Modern Nutrition Paul Pitchford, North Atlantic Books; 3 Rev Updated edition (February 28, 2003)

Articles:

1. Ben-Arye, E; Goldin, E; Wengrower, D; Stamper, A; Kohn, R; Berry, E (April 2002). "Wheat grass juice in the treatment of active distal ulcerative colitis: a randomized double-blind placebo-controlled trial". *Scand J Gastroenterol* **37** (4): 444–9. (http://dx.doi.org/10.1080%2F003655202317316088) . PMID 11989836 (http://www.ncbi.nlm.nih.gov/pubmed/11989836) .

2. Marawaha, RK; Bansal, D; Kaur, S; Trehan, A; Wheatgrass Juice Reduces Transfusion Requirement in Patients with Thalassemia Major: A Pilot Study. *Indian Pediatric* 2004 Jul;41(7):716-20

3. S. Mukhopadhyay; J. Basak; M. Kar; S. Mandal; A. Mukhopadhyay; Netaji Subhas; Chandra Bose; Cancer Research Institute, Kolkata, India; NRS Medical College,

Made in the USA
Las Vegas, NV
05 November 2021